Contents   **Page no.**

Nursing in secure environments

A scoping study conducted on behalf of the
United Kingdom Central Council
for Nursing, Midwifery and Health Visiting
by the Faculty of Health,
University of Central Lancashire

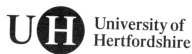
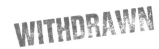

This report was written for, and not by, the UKCC.
The UKCC therefore accepts no responsibility for any
material inaccuracies or grammatical errors contained
within it and the individual views expressed are not
necessarily endorsed by the UKCC.

ISBN 1 901922 14 6

Foreword

Secure environments are amongst the most challenging arenas in which any registered nurse must work. Nurses provide services to clients within these environments in both the health services and the criminal justice system. This report was commissioned by the UKCC from the University of Central Lancashire in order to provide a comprehensive picture of the educational, occupational and practice expectations placed upon nurses working in secure environments across the United Kingdom.

The UKCC recognises the important role played by nurses in both the physical health care of clients and in the care and treatment of people with complex health and psychological needs. Nurses must balance the therapeutic needs of their clients with the security considerations demanded by society. In conducting the extensive research upon which this report is based, we have been impressed by the many examples of good practice which are delivering clear benefits, often under difficult circumstances, to clients in secure environments throughout the United Kingdom.

Secure mental health care and prison service policy has received considerable public attention in recent years and is likely to remain a major focus for health policy in the future. It is clear from this report that there are a number of issues which need to be addressed in order to ensure that all clients in secure environments are able to receive the highest possible standards of care. The UKCC has already determined its agenda for action arising from the University of Central Lancashire's report. Through this, we intend to work in partnership with registered nurses, policy makers and managers within the health and prison services to ensure that these issues are addressed quickly and decisively in order to provide the highest possible standards of care for clients in secure environments.

The UKCC commends the work undertaken by Les Storey and his colleagues at the University of Central Lancashire. A summary of this report and action plan has also been published by the UKCC and we will ensure that both reports receive the widest possible dissemination.

Alison Norman
UKCC President

November 1999

Overall Conclusions and Recommendations

Maintenance and monitoring of professional standards in secure settings relies on a joint approach by practitioners, managers of prison and health services, policy makers in the prison services and NHS, and statutory agencies.

Nurses working in the prison services and secure health settings remain accountable to the UKCC for their professional practice. The principles of clinical governance should underpin the development of health care provision in secure care and leadership in all of the services is a key method of ensuring that professional standards can be maintained and improved. Employers should support registered nurses to develop the necessary skills and approaches to prioritise, develop, monitor and audit standards.

The UKCC intends to integrate the findings from this report and issues raised during the dissemination of the findings into its current and future work programmes.

Recommendations

- The UKCC should ensure that the findings of this project be widely disseminated to key stakeholders. Such activity should also include the identification of any areas for future collaboration across the UK.

- The UKCC should take a proactive approach and engage key stakeholders in debate to ensure that they are aware of the importance of professional self-regulation in the maintenance of professional standards and high quality care in secure settings.

- The UKCC should actively encourage and support the development of nursing leadership and clinical supervision within secure environment services.

- The UKCC should ensure that the National Boards, education providers, education consortia/commissioners and other stakeholders are aware of the implications of the findings for education programmes (pre and post registration).

- The UKCC recommends that appropriate induction should always be provided for nurses working in secure care. Induction should be an integral part of a continuing professional development process that includes mentorship and clinical supervision.

- The UKCC recommends that there is due recognition and an evaluation of current service provision by the secure services of the needs of clients from all minority groups particularly those from ethnic minorities and women, to ensure that their health and other needs are identified and met in secure environments.

- The UKCC should collaborate with other appropriate agencies to take forward work on developing and improving professional standards (education and practice) in risk assessment, de-escalation and physical restraint of patients within secure environments. Collaborative work should also be undertaken to clarify professional practice issues and the maintenance of professional boundaries with clients in secure environments.

- The UKCC should explore with key stakeholders how good practice can be shared and the possibility of whether a UK-wide resource and dissemination centre might be established. The UKCC should enter into discussions about how research priorities and programmes might be affected by the outcomes of the project.

- The UKCC recommends that the secure services develop security policies to ensure that where there is an assessed health care need, patients should have access to appropriate healthcare services and that health care professionals should have ready access to patients to meet these identified needs.

- The UKCC recommends that in accordance with best practice in continuing professional development, practitioners continue to develop their knowledge and skills in order to monitor and meet the physical, psychological and security needs of patients on the basis of appropriate and comprehensive assessment.

- The UKCC recommends that the competency framework tested in this project should be validated by further work, and that the competencies be used to inform the design of nursing and midwifery roles, induction for those roles and continuous professional development.

1.0   Introduction

In its business plan for 1998/99 the Council identified the need to undertake a piece of work to scope issues involved in the work of practitioners working in secure environments. This work arose from a number of concerns including the rising number of calls and correspondence to the Council's Professional Advisory Service; concerns stimulated by the ongoing national inquiries into services in the mental health and prison services; concerns identified by senior nurses working within the secure environments field, and the need for Council to develop further its understanding and agenda in this area.

The scoping study represents the first time that the Council has comprehensively analysed the issues facing practitioners who work in secure environments. The outcomes of the work are expected to inform Council activity in standards and policy development for at least the next 5 years.

In July 1998 Council awarded a contract to the University of Central Lancashire to conduct a scoping study into nursing in secure environments.

The aim of the exercise was to provide a comprehensive overview of the educational, occupational and professional practice expectations placed on nurses working within secure environments. This would include both secure mental health services and Prison Services at all levels of security across the UK.

The objectives of the study were:

- describe the competencies required of nurses working in secure environments;
- assess whether nurses interventions in secure environments are evidence based;
- review current activity in the development of practice standards in secure environments, particularly with reference to specific client groups;
- review the effectiveness of the preparation currently given to nurses working in secure environments;
- identify issues faced in working with a client group who may compromise therapeutic nurse patient relationships, particularly with a reference to personality disordered patients;
- identify the extent to which existing Council policies are utilised and inform practice within secure environments; and
- identify practice issues relevant to the physical health needs of these populations; care of women (including care of pregnant women) and the care of people from different cultural backgrounds.

Since the commissioning of the work a number of UK and national policy initiatives have commenced which indicate that the work undertaken by the Council in scoping issues in secure environments is extremely timely. These include, amongst others: the reviews of mental health legislation in England and Wales, and Scotland; the publication of the *Future Organisation of Prison Health Care* in England, a major review of services for Mentally Disordered Offenders in Scotland; continued reporting by the Her Majesty's Inspectorates of Prisons of problems concerning health care delivery in prisons; recurring concerns stimulated by independent and public inquiries into service failures in mental health services; the England and Wales prison service review of principles and policy on mothers and babies in prison, and proposed Government policy initiatives on the care and treatment of those with personality disorder.

A steering group which met on 5 occasions and was supported by a project team at the University of Central Lancashire oversaw the project. The project was managed for the UKCC by the Professional Officer for Mental Health and Learning Disability, Richard Bradshaw and led for the University by Les Storey.

Unless otherwise stated, the 'Mental Health Act Commission' refers equally to the Mental Health Act Commission for England and Wales, the Mental Welfare Commission for Scotland and the Mental Health Commission for Northern Ireland.

Where reference is made to 'Mental Health Act', this refers equally to the Mental Health Act 1983 for England and Wales, the Mental Health (Scotland) Act 1984 and the Mental Health (Northern Ireland) Order 1986.

Unless otherwise stated, the term 'Prison Services' refers to Prison Services in England, Wales, Scotland and Northern Ireland.

2.0 The Development of Care in Secure Environments

Terminology

Nurses who work in Secure Environments in the United Kingdom provide a range of nursing services, and are represented on most parts of the UKCC Register. They are primarily employed by the Prison Services or by hospitals/health units in the NHS or private health care sector.

In the Prison Services, nurses meet the physical and mental health care needs of remanded and sentenced prisoners. The Prisons Services have a higher ratio of General Nurses than Mental Health Nurses, which reflects the services currently provided.

In the health sector nurses are primarily employed to meet the needs of people with mental health and/or learning disabilities, individuals physical health care is accommodated as far as possible within the hospital/unit's limitations.

Some nurses in the health sector are referred to as Forensic Nurses, which of itself is a term that causes confusion. Forensic is a word that is connected with the court, and in the health sector in the UK tends to imply that care is provided to mentally disordered offenders (MDOs). However, many of the patients within secure care have not offended and have not been in contact with the justice system. Some patients are placed in secure environments because of the danger they present either to themselves or others. Therefore the use of the title Forensic Nurse or Forensic Mental Health Nurse does not apply to all the nurses referred to in this scoping exercise.

Another area of confusion is the use of the term psychiatric in relation to nursing care. Registered Mental Nurses (RMNs) meet the needs of people with mental health problems, but if they work in the community they are referred to as Community Psychiatric Nurses (CPNs), and the organisation formed in 1987 by nurses working with MDOs, is the Forensic Psychiatric Nurses Association. The term's psychiatric and mental health tend to be used interchangeably within the profession, within the report they are used to reflect the context within which the terms are used.

International Perspectives on Forensic Nursing

Forensic nursing also has different connotations in different parts of the world, but appears to have two main forms, one type of forensic nurse deals with the victims of crime and the other deals with the perpetrator/offender.

In North America the term refers to nurses who deal with victims of crime. The International Association of Forensic Nurses (IAFN), which has members predominantly in the United States and Canada, defines forensic nursing as "the application of nursing science to public or legal proceedings: the application of the forensic aspects of health care combined with the bio-psycho-social education of the registered nurse in the scientific investigation and treatment of trauma and/or death of victims and perpetrators of abuse, violence, criminal activity and traumatic accidents" (IAFN 1999).

Forensic Nurses in North America fulfil some of the following roles as identified by Lynch (1993) and Evans and Wells (1999)

- Sexual Assault Nurse
- Nurse Coroner
- Nurse Investigator
- Forensic Psychiatric Nurse
- Forensic Correctional/Institutional Nurse
- Legal Nurse Consultant
- Nurse Attorneys
- Forensic Nursing Educators
- Forensic Gerontology Nurses
- Forensic Paediatric Nurses

Two of these roles, the Forensic Psychiatric Nurse and the Forensic Correctional Nurse reflect some of the roles undertaken by nurses working in Secure Environments in the United Kingdom. In the USA the Forensic Psychiatric Nurse was originally involved in assessing the mental state competency for persons charged with crimes (Lynch 1993, Coram 1993), as well as meeting the offenders care needs. The Correctional Nurse "cares for convicted criminals' physical health needs while incarcerated" (Coram 1993). Although as Evans and Wells (1999) state "Australian nurses working in forensic psychiatry hospitals would be more likely to call themselves forensic nurses although there is considerable confusion with the terms 'forensic' and 'correctional'. Additionally, in Australia, nurses working in forensic psychiatry hospitals would not necessarily see themselves as correctional nurses, but rather forensic psychiatric nurses". In Australia and New Zealand Forensic Nurses appear to fulfil a similar role, and encounter similar problems, to nurses in secure environments in the United Kingdom. Evans (1997) states that forensic nursing, in Australia is practised primarily in prisons and security hospitals nursing offenders/alleged offenders, whereas Carbonu and Soares (1997) provide an insight into forensic nursing in Pakistan, which provides support to the victims.

Although this scoping exercise is focusing on issues relating to nurses who work within a secure environment it is clear that these are not the only nurses providing forensic care. Evans and Bell (1999) cite an undated Royal College of Nursing document, from the UK, which lists the numerous locations in which forensic nurses provide care for mentally disordered offenders, these include: -

- Prisons
- Courts
- Police cells
- Social services establishments
- Generic community mental health settings
- Forensic community mental health settings
- Intensive therapy units
- Units for behaviourally disturbed people
- Units for those who are difficult to place

- Minimum (Low) Secure Units
- Forensic adolescent services
- High Security services- special hospitals
- Forensic independent sector provision

Many of these services are replicated throughout the world with slight variations. It is apparent from the literature that Forensic Nursing is developing a momentum and is becoming an area of specialism that is beginning to attract the attention it deserves, although the pace of change and the services provided vary in size and approach taken according to the needs of the countries involved.

2.1 The Development of Secure Hospital Care

High Security Provision

Since the eighteenth century Britain has had legislation controlling the activities of institutions for the mentally ill. An Act of 1763 ordered the segregation of "persons of insane mind and outrageous behaviour" (Donnelly 1983) and, in 1774 private madhouses were regulate under the Act for Regulating Madhouses (Chiswick 1993). The Vagrancy Acts of 1714 and 1744 also provided legislation to manage mentally disordered offenders. (McComish and Paterson 1996).

In Britain in 1800, James Hadfield was found not guilty by reason of insanity of an attempt to kill King George III, normally this would have resulted in his release, but because of his dangerousness he was returned to Newgate Prison (McComish and Paterson 1996). Shortly afterwards in the same year an Act 'for the safe custody of insane persons charged with offences' was passed by Parliament. This made statutory provision for the special verdict of not guilty by reason of insanity, and requiring the court to order the detention of the accused, following such a verdict, in strict custody until His Majesty's pleasure was known. (Kaye and Franey 1998)

This represents the origins of the present day concept of the hospital order and restriction order, and under the 1800 Act it became the Home Secretary's practice to order detention in Bethlem, where a special wing was built in 1815.

In 1843 the McNaughton case was another stage in the development of mental health legislation. McComish and Paterson (1996) relate the case of Daniel McNaughton who was tried for the wilful murder of the Prime Minister's, (Peel) Private Secretary (Drummond). McNaughton had suffered from delusions of persecution for a number of years; his complaints to his parents and the public authorities went unheeded so he devised a plan to kill Sir Robert Peel. The outcome of his trial for the murder of Drummond was that he was certified of unsound mind and detained in a lunatic asylum. This case caused uproar and the McNaughton Rules emerged, which were

- The defendant cannot be held responsible for his or her actions because of the severity of his or her mental illness. By reason of such defect from disease of the mind it is held that the defendant did not know the nature or the quality of his or her act (i.e. did not realise what he was physically doing at the time) Or
- By reason of such defect from the disease of the mind he or she did not know that the act was wrong (i.e. did not know that it was forbidden in law Or
- A person suffering from an insane delusion that prevents the appreciation of the nature and quality of the act has the same degree of responsibility as if the facts were as he or she imagined them

In 1856 the Home Secretary took the decision to build a new institution specially for the criminally insane. The Criminal Lunatics Act was passed in 1860 and Broadmoor opened in 1863. Thus the first English Special Hospital, Broadmoor came into existence serving the whole of England and Wales although the majority of criminal lunatics remained scattered across a variety of secure institutions until the 1870s.

Broadmoor soon reached its capacity and additional provision was commissioned. Initially this was provided in a temporary asylum at Parkhurst on the Isle of Wight, but permanent hospitals emerged at Rampton in 1912 and Moss Side in 1933.

In 1974, Park Lane Hospital opened on a site adjacent to Moss Side in two former Moss Side wards with a new hospital being built which opened in 1984. In 1990 Moss Side was formally amalgamated with the adjacent Park Lane Hospital to form Ashworth Hospital. In the process of reorganisation, the original Moss Side buildings were closed in 1995.

Direct Home Office management of Broadmoor ceased with the Criminal Justice Act 1948, when the term 'criminal lunatic' was abolished and the hospital management passed to the Board of Control. However, it remained solely for the use of mentally ill offenders, and admissions as well as discharges were the sole responsibility of the Home Secretary. It was not until the new legal arrangements established by the Mental Health Act 1959 and the Emery Report (Ministry of Health 1961) on the Special Hospitals, that the way was opened for the admission of patients under civil as well as criminal powers of detention.

Until 1989 the hospitals were administered directly by the Ministry of Health, when they became the responsibility of the Special Hospitals Service Authority. In 1996 each Special Hospital was created an Authority in its own right (similar to an NHS Trust) and a new purchasing body, the High Security Psychiatric Services Commissioning Board, was created as part of the NHS Executive. In 1999 the responsibility for commissioning High Secure services passed to the Regional Offices of the NHS Executive.

In Scotland, care of the mentally disordered offender was established in legislation as early as 1840 (Watson and Kirby 1999). Although, the Vagrancy Acts of 1714 and 1744 had provided a means for the disposal of mentally disordered offenders to local Bridewells and poor houses (McComish and Paterson 1996).

In the early 1800s great concern was expressed about Scottish prisons, they were felt to be entirely inappropriate for the disposal of criminal lunatics. These concerns led to the development of district asylums in Edinburgh, Dumfries, Glasgow and Aberdeen. In 1839 a bill was introduced to "improve prisons and prison discipline in Scotland" rather than providing a separate lunatic asylum in Scotland. In 1846 the laws on compulsory detention led to the development of the Criminal Lunatic Division of Perth Prison which became the predecessor to the State Hospital at Carstairs.

In 1952 the State Hospital opened on its current site and it joined the National Health Service as a Health Board.

The current philosophy of care and management for patients has evolved since a major incident in 1976 and the subsequent inquiry. Watson and Kirby (1999) suggest that the perceived success of The State Hospital, is due in part to the fact that they have less patients than the other High Secure Hospitals, and have introduced rigorous physical and relational security policies and protocols that reflect the needs not only of the patients but also the safety and security of the whole hospital community. The security systems and processes provide staff with an environment within which they can deliver therapy to meet the patients' needs.

In Northern Ireland there is no High or Medium Secure provision at present and the Province relies on Scotland to provide services. High Security is provided by the State Hospital at Carstairs, in Scotland, and Ashworth on Merseyside. A Regional Strategy is being developed in an attempt to provide a Medium Secure Unit in the Province by 2002.

Medium Secure/Regional Services

Over the last 20 years other forensic psychiatry systems have developed. Regional forensic psychiatry services based on regional/medium secure units, which are small and integrated with local psychiatric and social services, and low secure provision within NHS Trusts.

The concept of Medium Secure Unit provision originated in 1957 when the report of the Royal Commission proposed that dangerous patients should be accommodated in a few hospitals having suitable facilities for their treatment and custody. In 1959, the then Minister of Health, Enoch Powell, appointed a working party to consider the provision of security in psychiatric hospitals and Special Hospitals: it reported in July 1961.

By the 1960s it was apparent that the open door policy of mental hospitals and the wholly commendable trend towards voluntary rather than compulsory admission to hospital for psychiatric treatment, was resulting in the neglect of a certain section of the mentally disordered population. The Special Hospitals providing for treatment of patients in conditions of maximum security were very overcrowded. Patients were being detained in those hospitals for longer than was necessary. Faced with increasing numbers of such people ending up in prison, there were two reports commissioned in the early 1970s. One into secure provision in the NHS (The Glancy Report 1974) and the other more widely targeting all aspects of the problems posed to society by the mentally abnormal offender (The Butler Report 1974).

The Glancy Report recommended immediate planning for 1,000 secure beds at regional level, a formula approximating to 20 beds per million of the catchment population, whilst 4 months later the Butler Committee (1974) published an interim report stressing the urgency of providing regional secure units. They described a yawning gap between NHS hospitals with no secure provision and the overcrowded Special Hospitals, although there was some provision in psychiatric hospitals for patients remanded for reports, patients on section 60, transfers from prisons and for patients who might have been transferred to Special Hospitals.

In 1976 the first Interim Secure Units were opened, but it was not until November 1980 that the first Regional/Medium Secure Unit began admitting patients and it then took over 2½ years for a further 3 units to open. They were intended to be well staffed and accommodate patients whose length of stay was not intended to exceed two years (The Butler Report 1974).

In Scotland, the strategy for secure mental health is based on the principles outlined in the Reed Report (Department of Health 1992). The implementation of the Framework for Mental Health Services in Scotland will result in a range of in-patient facilities that will include forensic services integrated with mainstream Mental Health Services, in an attempt to decrease stigmatism. The Framework also recommends that national standards for service provision, qualifications and competencies for nurses, particularly in relation to the use of Cognitive Behaviour Therapies, should be developed (Scottish Office 1999).

In Northern Ireland, the development of Medium Secure provision has been debated for a number of years. In the late 1970's, a site was identified at Purdysburn, now renamed the Knockbracken Health Care Park, to build an MSU. Browne (1999) reports that in 1984 the DHSS for Northern Ireland published *Mental Health -The Way Forward*, the Report of the Review Committee on services for the mentally ill. The report welcomed "the development of psychiatric resources within the Prison Medical Service and consider that they should be further developed to the extent required to cope as far as possible with all mentally ill prisoners" but went on to say that "In view of the general attitude of staff and the small number of patients that require periods of accommodation in a secure environment we do not think that the substantial initial capital and annual running costs associated with a Medium Secure Unit could not be justified. We therefore suggest that intensive care units should be developed at each hospital and within existing accommodation."

In 1994 the issue was re-opened in the Joint DHSS Northern Ireland Office working parties recommendation to develop an MSU and comprehensive Forensic Service including outreach services (Browne 1999. This development is outlined in the Department of Health and Social Services' strategy in which the preferred site suggested is the Knockbracken Health Care Park, the old Purdysburn Hospital. A Regional Inter-agency group is being established to look at the implications for developing these services, priorities will include:

- In patient services
- Community Residential Forensic Rehabilitation
- Police and Court liaison
- Prison Services
- Forensic Community services and liaison
- Forensic Psychotherapy services.

Levels of Provision

Within the health sector, secure environments are provided for patients who have mental health problems or learning disabilities. Secure environments are provided at low, medium and high levels within the appropriate mental health legislation for England and Wales (Mental Health Act 1983), The Mental Health (Scotland) Act 1984, and The Mental Health (Northern Ireland) Act 1986. The legislation is fundamentally parallel across the four countries.

High Security

Three High Secure Hospitals in England and the State Hospital in Scotland offer a range of therapeutic services similar to those provided in ordinary psychiatric hospitals but in conditions of greater security. Patients in these hospitals are predominantly those who have come into contact with the criminal justice system and are remanded in custody or have been convicted and enter the sentenced prison population. In England, Mentally disordered people in prison can be transferred to the NHS under the Mental Health Act 1983 using Section 47 (for sentenced prisoners) and section 48 (for remand prisoners); similar legislation is in force in Scotland, Wales and Northern Ireland. One of the dilemmas identified for hospital staff is the small group of individuals who are transferred into secure health care after serving the bulk of their prison sentence. These patients close to their earliest date of release (EDR) can present as being angry and de-motivated when transferred into these settings.

In England, the National Health Service Act 1977 (Section 7) requires the Secretary of State to Provide Special (High Secure) Hospitals for detained mentally disordered patients "who in his opinion require treatment under conditions of special security on account of their dangerousness, violent or criminal propensities".

When considering an application for a patient to be admitted to a High Secure Hospital there are three main criteria to be met:

1. The presence or absence of a recognisable mental disorder, i.e. mental illness, psychopathic disorder, mental impairment or severe mental impairment and any other disorder or disability of mind
2. Whether that individual presents as a grave and immediate danger to the public
3. Whether (in relation to severe mental impairment, mental impairment or psychopathic disorder) that person will be amenable to treatment.

Medium Security

Medium/Regional Secure Units increased significantly between 1991 and 1995. There are now an estimated 2,600 beds available in these units. "The term 'Medium Secure Unit' is used interchangeably in the contemporary field with Regional Secure Unit. More correctly, the term RSU appertains to NHS provided medium secure units, whereas the term MSU applies to any unit, NHS or independent sector, that offers medium levels of security". (Tarbuck 1996)

The target group is patients who are too difficult or dangerous to be managed in local hospitals but who do not require the security available at the High Secure Hospitals. Medium Secure beds are intended for fairly short-term use, around 18 months, and cannot cater for those with longer term needs. The Department of Health has defined medium (or regional) security as being for "those who require specialised care and treatment in wards or units offering care in conditions of greater security than that available in local locked wards, but less than that in high security". (Department of Health 1992a)

Low Security

Low security beds, such as locked wards in general psychiatric hospitals are currently provided for short term treatment of intensively ill people; slow stream treatment, and rehabilitation for people with challenging behaviour; long term care for people with treatment resistant illness. These beds are provided for those people who present some risk to themselves or others would leave the premises without permission, but who are unlikely to attempt to use force to achieve this (Mental Health Foundation 1997). Discussions with participants in the scoping exercise suggest that the availability of services at this level are insufficient to meet current and anticipated needs.

It has not been easy to establish an exact picture of establishments that provide secure environments in the health sector because different assumptions about levels of security are made by health service organisations. However, from data gathered from The Forensic Directory (Rampton Hospital Authority 1998) and Regional Offices of the NHS Executive the numbers of organisations in the public and private sectors of health care appears to be as follows:

Level of Security	High	Medium	Low
Number of Establishments	4	38	96

Patient Characteristics

The patients who reside in the range of secure units throughout the country are a very disparate group with a wide range of needs. Patients with mental health problems include adults who

- have not committed an offence but whose behaviour brings them to the attention of the police;
- have not committed an offence but whose illness or behaviour leads to their being detained under the Mental Health Acts, sometimes in secure facilities
- have committed a minor offence but whose primary need is for mental health services and whom it is not in the public interest to detain or prosecute
- have committed an offence and who will be prosecuted but whose mental health problems are such that a prison sentence would be an inappropriate disposal; they require treatment in a secure psychiatric hospital
- have committed an offence and who will be prosecuted and may then enter the prison population with a mental health problem;
- develop a mental health problem whilst in prison

Other patients are detained because they are "unfit to plead", "insane on arraignment", or "at Her Majesty's pleasure"

In considering the needs of those patients detained in secure health facilities the latest statistics available from the Home Office were examined (Issue 19/98, 25 September 1998, Statistics of Mentally Disordered Offenders in England and Wales 1997 by Kershaw and Renshaw).

This bulletin provides information about patients subject to a restriction order (restricted patients) admitted to, detained in or discharged from hospitals in England and Wales:

- The number in hospital at the end of 1997 was 2,694. This was 6 per cent more than the previous year, similar to the average yearly increase in recent years.
- The number admitted under hospital orders fell from 243 in 1996 to 211 in 1997, while the number recalled to hospital rose from 74 to 100. The number transferred from prison to hospital remained the same, at 745, as the previous year.
- The total number admitted to hospitals was 1,074 in 1997. This was 5 fewer than the previous year.

- The number of restricted patients released into the community increased between 1996 and 1997 from 321 to 333.

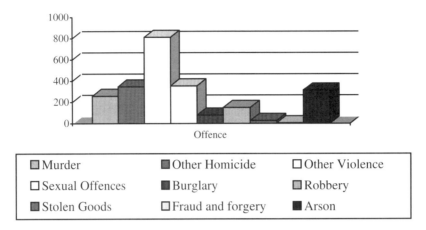

Restricted Patients Detained in Hospital by Offence (England & Wales, 31

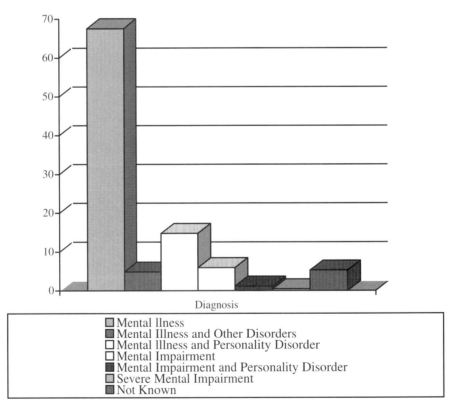

Dec.1997)Restricted Patients Detained in Hospital by Type of Mental Disorder
Source: Home Office (1998)

Between 1987 and 1997 admissions of restricted patients to hospital almost trebled from 385 to 1,074 patients. The number of admissions grew to a peak in 1994 (1,117) and has since fluctuated a little below this level. The overall figure for transfers from prison to hospital rose more than threefold between 1989 and 1993, but has remained relatively stable since. Also notable during this time frame has been the growth in health beds for mentally disordered offenders outwith the High Security (Special Hospitals). In 1987 there was a total of 1,172 patients in High Security hospitals in England and Wales this total has remained relatively consistent through until 1997 when the figure is recorded as 1,203. In 'Other Hospitals' however the numbers of detained patients has risen incrementally from 656 in 1987 to 1,491 in 1997.

As in previous years, most restricted patients detained in hospital at the end of 1997 were diagnosed as having a mental illness (with or without other disorders) – 72%. An additional 16 per cent were diagnosed as suffering from some form of psychopathic disorder.

Between 1987 and 1997 the proportion of restricted patient admissions who were suffering from mental illness (with or without other disorders) increased from 79 per cent to 92 per cent. This was mainly due to the large increase over this period in the proportion of hospital admissions transferred from prison. Conversely, the proportion of patients admitted suffering from a psychopathic disorder fell from 12 per cent in 1987 to 4 per cent in 1997.

Among admissions in 1997, the largest single groups (some 39 per cent) were those convicted of, or charged with, acts of violence against the person, including homicide. However, the proportion has fallen from 58 per cent in 1987. The number of restricted patients admitted having been convicted of, or having been charged with, sexual offences has grown from 36 in 1987 to 92 in 1997, although the proportions have remained relatively stable. Admissions for burglary increased from 25 in 1987 to 101 in 1997, while those for robbery grew from 32 to 107. The proportion of patients admitted for either burglary or robbery increased from 14 per cent in 1987 to 19 per cent in 1997.

In 1997, the number of patients aged 21 to 39 admitted to hospital (766) accounted for 71 per cent of total admissions. Among patients aged 40 or over, violence against the person and sexual offences were more common than in the younger age group, with far fewer committing robbery or burglary. Those suffering from a psychopathic disorder were convicted of or charged with proportionately the highest number of violent offences of those admitted in 1997 (47 per cent). Sexual offences were more common among the small number with a mental impairment or severe mental impairment (6 out of 24 admissions).

Among restricted patients detained in hospital at the end of 1997, 53 per cent (1,415) had been convicted of, or charged with, acts of violence against the person. In 257 of these cases the offence was murder and in 347 it was other homicide. 13 per cent of the restricted population had been convicted of, or charged with, sexual offences and 12 per cent arson. Among the sentenced population violent offences were the most common for patients suffering from mental illness, while sexual offences accounted for the highest proportion of offences for those with mental impairment.

Ethnic Minorities in General and Forensic Psychiatry

The term ethnic minority is used currently to identify people whose origins lie outside the United Kingdom, but more specifically, it is used for people of African, Afro-Caribbean or Asian origin (McNaught, 1987).

During an eighteen-month period between 1992 and 1994, a task force appointed by the NHS Executive consulted with African-Caribbean and Asian communities about their experiences of mental health services under the government's community care policies (Department of Health, 1994). This survey showed that: (a) African-Caribbeans, including large numbers of women, continue to be over-represented in psychiatric institutions at all levels; (b) psychiatric treatment often does not take account of the impact of race and racism; (c) there is no widespread acceptance of the importance of culturally diverse methods in working with black mental health users and carers; and (d) general practitioners (GPs) fail to respond adequately to black clients' complaints, leading to crisis admissions and compulsory admissions in medium secure units with treatment involving high drug dosages. The result of all this is that: (1) in practice, black people access mental health services at a much later stage than those in the general population, necessitating crisis and, therefore, controlling responses; (2) because of the nature of societal attitudes concerning race and crime, there is a high probability that black people will be taken into the criminal justice system; and (3) once they get there, and are deemed to be in mental distress or suffering from mental ill health, because of the ways in which their cultures, actions and mores may be interpreted or mis-interpreted, they are more likely to be given more punitive disposals at the severe end of psychiatric treatment.

This over representation of people from ethnic minorities in the western psychiatric system has been a problem identified for some considerable time. Ranney (1850) claimed that immigrants were "disappointingly represented" in American asylums.

Diagnosis

Studies based on hospital admissions (Carpenter and Brockington, 1980; Dean Walsh and Downing, 1981; Rwegellera, 1977) show an increased overall rate of mental disorder among West Indians; with schizophrenia being the commonest diagnosis. Adebimpe (1981) suggests that black patients run a higher risk of being misdiagnosed than white patients are. They may be over-diagnosed in one area and under-diagnosed in another. The diagnosis of schizophrenia is experienced by most black people as a tool for their oppression and control rather than for the alleviation of their suffering and the promotion of their well being (Fernando, Ndegwoo and Wilson, 1998).

The Transcultural Psychiatry Society has estimated that at least 40,000 Afro-Caribbean's will be misdiagnosed at least once in their lives because GPs and psychiatrists are inadequately trained to recognise their symptoms (Doku, 1990).

Admissions

Admissions statistics in the UK from the 1980's show that Afro-Caribbeans continued to be more likely to be admitted to mental institutions than native-born white people (Mercer,

1986). Of particular concern is the overrepresentation of Afro-Caribbeans as recipients of enforced incarceration under Section 136 of the Mental Health Act subsequent to police referrals (Rogers and Faulkner, 1987) and many studies reveal misdiagnosis and racial stereotyping (Shasidharan, 1988). Francis (1996) notes that, "young black men are the most feared sector of our population and their predicament commands a disproportionate amount of attention by the media". Which concurs with Farrington (1993) that, "There is a well established stereotype of the black psychiatric patient as volatile and dangerous".

Agbolegbe (1991) reported that black people are proportionally over-represented in mental hospitals in the UK. They are five times more likely to receive custodial (often-enforced) treatment, and twice as likely to have their first diagnosis changed, to see junior staff and to receive physical treatment rather than psychological therapy. Farrington (1993) described the provision of mental health services for ethnic minorities in the 1980s and early 1990s as "haphazard and inconsistent".

The Department of Health (1992) established a specific sub group under the review of services for mentally disordered offenders to consider the issue of ethnic minorities. They reported that, "Studies over the past 20 years show that black people who come to the attention of psychiatric services are more likely than white people to be:

- removed by the police to a place a safety under Section 136 of the Mental Health Act 1983;
- detained in hospital under Sections 2, 3 and 4 of the Mental Health Act;
- diagnosed as suffering from schizophrenia or other form of psychotic illness;
- be detained in locked wards of psychiatric hospitals;
- receive higher dosages of medication.

They are less likely than white people to:
- receive appropriate and acceptable diagnosis or treatment for possible mental illness at an early stage;
- receive treatments such as psychotherapy or counselling.

The report goes on to suggest that 'A number of studies have shown that patients from minority ethnic communities receive an inferior or discriminatory service with "stereotyping" being common'. The Mental Health Act Commission (1991) in its 4th Biennial Report commented (para 3.6(e) iii) that "many professionals seemed to lack basic knowledge about the different needs of ethnic minority communities and to have little real understanding of institutional racism and the effect of cultural difference on the nature of mental disorder."

McKenzie (1999) in his recent editorial in the British Medical Journal argues that institutional racism, "goes to the very core of health care practice", and that in the area of health he identified several consequences of institutional racism. "People from minority ethnic communities have poorer health, poorer access to services, and are treated differently, especially in psychiatry".

Secure Care and Ethnic Issues

A study of compulsorily detained patients at the Maudsley Hospital (Moodley and Thornicroft, 1988) showed that all the West Indian patients were detained in locked wards

23

at the time of admission, compared with half of the white men. Furthermore, medication was more likely to be administered immediately to black than to white detained patients. In a study in Nottingham (Chen Harrison and Standon, 1991) showed that a depot injection was more likely to be given to African-Caribbean's than to other ethnic groups; and it was also given earlier in the course of treatment. Seclusion was used more commonly for black patients (compared to whites) at a US University hospital (Soloff and Turner, 1981). This was explained by the researchers as resulting from attribution to black patients of violent traits, cultural prejudice, fear and distrust ... compromising the quality of understanding between patient and staff and contributing ultimately to a system of bias in seclusion practice (1981:43).

In 1995 the Department of Health ran a series of regional seminars on "Black Mental Health" (Department of Health, 1995) and reported that many participants, across all communities, point to racism as having a pervasive effect on the lives of black people. Two points were predominant:

1) many black people regard racism and its effects as a major contributing factor in the mental ill health of black people.

2) the view is that the needs of black people can be overlooked.

Fernando, Ndegwoo and Wilson (1998) concur with this view and state that, "There is no doubt that racism adversely affects the mental health of black people. The consequence for many black people with mental health problems, particularly those who encounter forensic psychiatry, is that they are at the mercy of a system which neither knows their real needs (because they have remained largely invisible), nor in the main, understands the importance of, or need, to explore ways of meeting them in a fundamental way".

They go on to state that:

- The special hospitals have been the subject of much criticism not least on account of their failure to address issues of human rights, racial discrimination and mistreatment of women.

- Although there has been no published ethnic statistics on the use of restriction orders by courts, it is obvious (and verified by unpublished research) that black people (as compared to white people) are disproportionately over-represented.

- Forensic psychiatry colludes with images of dangerousness and fear associated with black people

In their current review of mental health services in the UK the Standing Nursing and Midwifery Committee (SNMAC) state that, "In all aspects of the work we have carried out themes connected with the racial and cultural diversity in our society have become apparent. There is clear dissatisfaction from users and carers from minority ethnic and racial groups concerning access to services, satisfaction with services provided, and appropriate involvement of various racial and cultural groups in the planning, delivery and evaluation of care."(SNMAC, 1999)

The lack of basic knowledge about the needs of minority ethnic communities and poor understanding of institutional racism noted by the Mental Health Act Commission raises questions about how the differing needs of minority communities are met in hospital. It does not appear that consideration has often been given to the relationship between the alleged lack of co-operation by the patient and lack of knowledge and understanding by the staff.

All patients require access to a complaints procedure in which they have confidence. The Mental Health Act Commission has expressed doubts that this exists for patients from ethnic communities. Some commissioners have observed that black patients tend to regard racist attitudes of staff as a normal experience of institutional life that does not qualify as a matter for complaint (4th Biennial Report: Mental Health Act Commission, 1991).

A number of studies have shown that Afro-Caribbean patients are found in conditions of higher security than white. Cope (1989) found that the rate for young Afro-Caribbean's detained under Part 111 of the Mental Health Act was twenty-five times higher than the white rate, with a larger number of Afro-Caribbean's likely to receive restriction orders. The MHAC 8th Biennial Report (1997-1999) states that , "the use of the (Mental Health) Act for Black ethnic groups is 6 times greater than the proportion of such groups in the population as a whole, while the use for Asian groups is roughly in line with their presence in the general population". (MHAC 1999).

Edwards (1992) notes that the consequent disadvantage which frames black people's experiences within the context of forensic psychiatry occurs for a number of reasons: First, because labels, stereotypes and images associated with black people engender fear, misunderstanding and an accompanying tendency to react repressively; second, because there is frequently little common ground or understanding between, on the one hand, the major players in both the criminal justice system (police officers, magistrates, probation officers) and the mental health system (consultant psychiatrists, social workers, community psychiatric nurses) and, on the other, black people; third, because black people are viewed as having no part in the shaping of the current system of justice in Britain and fourth, because the interface between black communities and the police, governed by suspicion and a lack of knowledge, results in black people being more likely to be "stopped, searched, arrested, charged, convicted and to receive a custodial sentence than white people" (Edwards, 1992).

Browne (1990), in an exploratory study into the psychiatric remand process as it affects black defendants at magistrates courts, concluded that "coupled with magistrates lack of experience and unfamiliarity with the provisions of the 1983 Mental Health Act, and the unavoidably subjective nature of decisions, they are expected to make ... decisions are not always made in the best medical interests of mentally disturbed defendants generally, and black defendants in particular" (1990: 28). At the other end of the scale, evidence suggests that black people's access to psychiatric services via their general practitioners is considerably less than that of their counterparts in the larger community (Wilson, 1993; Department of Health, 1994).

The issues noted in general psychiatric services about security, high dosages of medication and lack of sensitivity to racial and cultural issues are equally applicable. The Mental

Health Act Commission has commented in its 4th Biennial Report on displays of racist material in a special hospital.

Staffing and training in relation to ethnic minorities

Considerable comment has been made about the very low number of management and professional staff from minority ethnic communities in senior positions in the health service and throughout the criminal justice system and social services. Most agencies and professionals have begun to address these issues and a number have introduced equal opportunities policies for users and staff (Department of Health, 1992; SNMAC, 1999). Bilingual staff, as well as skilled and qualified interpreters are also in short supply (Fernando Ndegwoo and Wilson, 1998). Black staff working in institutions where the ethos is predominantly 'white' often face considerable problems in having their views heard, quite apart from being acted upon (Fernando, 1996; Wilson, 1998).

In their recent review of Mental Health Nursing the Standing Nursing and Midwifery Advisory Committee (SNMAC 1999) comment that, "There is a consensus that the uptake of the recommendation no. 35 of Working in Partnership (i.e. that education and training programmes reflect the way that diversity of belief systems and cultural expectations contribute to the life experience of people who use services), has been patchy to say the least". Involvement by members of various minority ethnic and racial groups is often non-existent in the planning, teaching and evaluation of educational programmes.

However, anti-racist training of staff working in forensic psychiatry together with strongly enforced anti-racist policies may go some way towards redressing some of the injustice that prevails in the operation of forensic psychiatry (Fernando Ndegwoo and Wilson, 1998). There is a consensus that there is considerable variation in the awareness of staff to issues of race and culture across inpatient mental health services. In turn, practices relating to race and culture are extremely variable (SNMAC 1999).

The training of staff who work in British forensic services seldom adequately addresses issues of race and cultural difference (Doku, 1990). Agbolegbe (1991) states that, "Evidence suggests that professionals be they doctors, nurses or social workers, solicitors policemen or psychiatrists are not trained to be responsive to the needs of a changed and a changing society".

Despite guidance from the Home Office and the Department of Health racist practices persist and place black people with some degree of mental disorder in a particularly vulnerable position. It is therefore of key importance that services are developed which are sensitive to symptoms of mental distress and which can offer appropriate help at an early stage.

The lack of understanding and knowledge about race and culture, euro-centric assumptions, and the racist attitudes of some of those involved in the various services are a common theme from the literature. All authorities agree that professional education should take account of issues of race and culture and that all agencies should identify staff training needs and establish programmes.

A considerable need for research has been identified. Issues include: compulsory detention under the Mental Health Act; the diagnosis of schizophrenia; the views of ethnic minorities of the psychiatric services; the care and treatment provided to ethnic minorities in hospital; the services provided in the community; issues around the decision-making process of the Crown Prosecution Service and the courts; diversion from custody; and the role of the police.

Treatment Needs of Mentally Disordered Offenders

Maden *et al.* (1995) considered the "Treatment and Security Needs of Special Hospital Patients" and in doing so attempted to compare and contrast their needs with patients at other levels of security in the health sector. Their research concluded, "The clinical teams were much more optimistic about the chances of moving patients on to less secure settings than about improvement in the patient's clinical condition. The clinical teams see their task as one of rehabilitation, minimising secondary and tertiary handicaps, rather than an attempt to 'cure' the original disorder. Nevertheless, the prevalence of treatment-resistant psychosis suggests a huge potential demand for any new drug treatment."

They went on to suggest that it was difficult to identify other patient characteristics that distinguished the 'maximum secure' and the 'medium secure' patients within their sample. The diagnoses were similar, although the 'maximum secure' group contained an excess of patients with sexual disorders. Patients with learning disabilities were more likely to receive a lower security rating but there has been a decrease in the number of patients with this diagnosis in the Special Hospitals over the past few years and many of those who remain could not easily be placed elsewhere. The team stated that, "The point emerging from many of these tables is that the distinction between patients needing maximum or medium security is not easy to pin down. It is a matter of degree or judgement, rather than a clear, qualitative difference, in most cases"(Maden *et al* 1995).

It was also difficult from the Maden *et al.* (1995) research to find clinical features to distinguish diagnostic groups within their sample. There were some obvious differences but the range of clinical problems and treatment needs of patients with very different diagnoses were often very similar. "This does not mean that the population is homogeneous; there is a vast range of problems and treatment needs within it but neither diagnosis nor security need was a good predictor of these differences".

The list of perceived obstacles to discharge or transfer from the Maden *et al.* (1995) study shows few marked differences between the different levels of security. The list is headed by the same problems: lack of understanding of the offence by the patient, difficulty relating to others and lack of response to medication. Only around 10% of patients are considered an absconding risk.

Maden *et al* (1995) compiled a list of issues that were indicated by the patients' clinical teams as determining a need for security and presenting as potential obstacles to discharge or transfer:

- Offence not understood by patient
- Difficulty relating to others
- Lack of response to medication

- Likely non-co-operation with supervision
- Likely non-compliance with medication
- Alcohol or drug abuse
- Current aggression
- Current non-compliance with medication
- Lack of co-operation with staff
- Index offence not understood by team
- Absconding risk in lesser security
- Current self-harm
- Non co-operation with psychotherapy

The description of therapeutic needs is also consistent across the security levels and is dominated by nursing care, occupational therapy and medication.

Patients identified by clinical team as having current therapeutic needs:

- Nursing care (next 12 months)
- Occupational therapy
- Medication
- Escorted Leave
- Individual Psychotherapy (in next 5 years)
- Nursing Care (for next 5 years)
- Behavioural Treatments
- Interaction with opposite sex
- Sexual assessment
- Group psychotherapy

Mental Health Policy Development and its Impact on Forensic Services

The process of de-institutionalisation has led to changes in both the in-patient population and the settings in which care takes place. In-patient care now largely takes place in the wards of district general hospital psychiatric units, although some wards remain in older mental hospitals. Hospital admissions are of much shorter duration than they were, and many patients who used to be treated in hospital are now treated in the community, leading to higher levels of acuity in the hospital in-patient population.

The in-patient population is now largely composed of people with serious and enduring mental illness, such as schizophrenia and mood disorder. A great deal of evidence suggests in-patients have greater levels of disadvantage, social exclusion, homelessness, and a much wider and more complex set of needs than they did in the past. For example, the number of patients who have problems both with substance abuse and/or dependence and a mental illness has risen steeply. Patients with co-morbidity place great demands on the clinical skills of nurses, who are often not trained to provide the complexity of care that they require.

SNMAC(1999) cited several reports have expressed disquiet about the environment in acute psychiatric facilities. Working in Partnership (Department of Health 1994) recommended that there be an urgent review of the therapeutic suitability of district general hospital mental health units. Meanwhile, there is concern that patients often do not have privacy, nor are they guaranteed the therapeutic and recreational facilities that are a necessary part of good care. There is clear evidence that women are particularly disadvantaged with regard to both privacy and safety.

The current Government legislative framework includes 'The new NHS' and "Towards a Healthier Scotland" which spell out the need for health services to tackle the root causes of ill health, ensure high standards of health care, and quicker treatment. In England, *Modernising Social Services* (DSS 1998) highlights three priorities for personal social services: promoting independence, improving protection, and raising standards. Both the NHS and Social Services are charged to work more in partnership to provide integrated services that will improve the quality of life for the population.

Government strategies for mental health services in the new millennium are set out in the *Framework for Mental Health Services in Scotland* (Scottish Office 1997), and in *Modernising Mental Health Services: Safe, Sound and Supportive* (Department of Health 1998) (the policy framework for Northern Ireland is set out in a separate paper but has fundamentally similar aims and objectives but no position has been articulated for Wales).

The laws on mental health are being reviewed-date across the United Kingdom: in particular, to ensure that patients who might otherwise be a danger to themselves and others are no longer allowed to refuse to comply with the treatment they need. The law will be changed to permit the detention of a small group of people who have not committed a crime but whose untreatable psychiatric disorder makes them dangerous, either to themselves or others.

Specific developments include 24 hour crisis teams to respond to emergencies, more acute mental health beds, more hostels and supported accommodation, more home treatment teams, more training for all involved in dealing with patients who are mentally ill and access to NHS Direct for 24 hour help and advice.

The National Institute for Clinical Excellence and a Clinical Standards Advisory Group, in England, and the Clinical Standards Board for Scotland, are being established. Together with the development of National Service Frameworks for mental health, they will ensure that clear and authoritative guidance is available on the most effective drugs and therapies. Action is already being taken to improve mental health services for young people. The National Service Framework for Older People will consider the mental health needs of older people.

The Government has acknowledged that unacceptable variations in performance and practice continue. They also acknowledge that people with mental health problems often have complex needs which cross traditional organisational and professional boundaries and that substance misuse or personality disorder make treatment of mental illness more difficult.

Specific areas identified include the complex areas of child and adolescent psychiatry, meeting the needs of women and addressing issues of co-morbidity.

The Government strategies seek to address the issue of bed shortage by ensuring that there are enough beds of the right kind in the right place. This will include "the whole range including 24 hour staffed beds, acute beds, and secure beds to make sure that pressures do not build up in any one part of the system". (Department of Health 1999).

The Government strategy states that patients who present a risk to others sometimes need to be looked after in secure accommodation, where they can receive the care and help they need. A shortage of locally available secure beds can mean that some patients are cared for in acute psychiatric wards, further adding to pressures in the system. The Government proposes to provide extra secure places to ensure the whole care system works together to provide, "the right care in the right place at the right time".

The Government states that it is determined to improve the quality and accessibility of secure hospital services. At present, there are too many cases where people who need secure care cannot be found a bed, remaining inappropriately placed in secure wards or prisons for far too long. This situation is partly a consequence of the continued separation of both commissioning and provision of high security services from the arrangements that apply to other NHS secure mental health services, and the limited role of commissioners in evaluating the needs of individuals within the prison population.

In line with its policy on Social Inclusion, the Government has stated its intention to improve the way that people with a severe personality disorder are managed, particularly in cases where they present a grave risk to the public. Most people in this group who are convicted of offences are sentenced to a term of imprisonment. Some are admitted to psychiatric hospital if their personality disorder is recognised and judged to be treatable. But, currently the law requires that people with a severe personality disorder may be released at the end of a prison sentence or discharged from hospital even though they still present a significant risk.

There is also a small group of people with severe personality disorder who come to the attention of mental health or social services practitioners, or to the police, as presenting a genuine risk but who have not been involved in any criminal offence. "People in this group may benefit from a range of interventions intended to reduce risk, but not all are suitable for treatment as patients in hospital settings. These people fall outside the scope of the Mental Health Act and cannot be detained or required to comply with supervision". (Department of Health 1998)

The Government is therefore considering proposals to create a new form of reviewable detention for those people with a severe personality disorder who are considered to pose a grave risk to the public. The principles the Government is adopting in working up these proposals are as follows:

- the safety of the public is of prime concern;
- admission to the new regime will not be dependent upon the person having committed an offence, nor whether they are treatable under the terms of the current Mental Health Act;
- release into the community will depend upon a rigorous assessment that the person no longer poses a grave risk to the public;

- the regime will comply with the Government's obligε
  Human Rights.

The proposals are likely to require the development of speciε
with a dangerous severe personality disorder, under conditions
security and interventions designed to reduce and manage their rι
by some authors, including Prins and Swan (1998), as a respons
accuse the government of arbitrary policy decisions, which are "m
political expediency, driven by public concerns over care in the comnι
cause celebres. The notoriety of the case seeming to be more due to ι.
alarming nature than to the intrinsic merit of the facts" (Prins and Swan 1ϧ

The Government proposals set out in Managing Dangerous People with Severe Personality Disorder (Home Office 1999) suggests options for the management of this group which will influence the way nurses develop in the future.

Forensic Mental Health Nursing

Forensic nursing takes place across a broad range of care settings from community to high secure hospitals with its many pressing legal, political and multi-professional priorities. In the midst of so many considerations, nursing has barely had a voice and has struggled for recognition within the context of more powerful and perhaps informed professional agendas. Consequently, no formal theoretical framework, accommodating the interface between nursing roles and forensic patients' psychopathologies exists and no adequate formulation about what needs to be "special" about forensic nursing over and above providing, empathic, empowering care for stigmatised populations under difficult conditions has been developed either. (Aiyegbusi 1997)

The role of the mental health nurse has changed radically in recent years. In 1968, when the first review of mental health nursing entitled Psychiatric Nursing Today and Tomorrow (1968) was published there were approximately 130,000 in-patients mostly housed in old Victorian asylums. By 1994, the second review of mental health nursing, Working in Partnership (1994) there were only 25,000 in-patient beds and numbers have continued to declined.

Forensic psychiatric nursing is described as a specialist branch of psychiatric nursing. (Robinson and Kettles 1998; Morrison and Burnard 1992). Morrison and Burnard also acknowledge the lack of clarity and research associated with "the cloud of confusion that currently hovers over the field of forensic psychiatric nursing". These observations about forensic psychiatric nursing seem to reflect a curious though enduring "split" whereby there is a hint of "specialist" expertise on one hand while lack of definition and theoretical frameworks, or indeed a recognised clinical practice base exist on the other.

The difficulties that have plagued inquiries into forensic services have taken little account of the psychodynamic interplay between patients and staff of all disciplines and backgrounds, within the closed environments of secure environments (Duffy, Clifton and Dale 1997).

The patients' mental disorder and offending poses intense demands upon nurses because of that they maintain empathic and objective relationships while remaining in the patients' prior offending in order to retain a focus on risk.

In a recent publication, Killian and Clark (1996) begin to explore some of the more complex interpersonal issues associated with nursing in forensic services. These authors describe the challenges associated with applying humanistic interventions instead of more mechanistic ones in forensic nursing.

The exchange of physical boundaries for the security provided by relationships that patients develop with nurses, places a large demand upon nursing staff. They have to provide emotional and practical (physical) containment whilst allowing at the same time, for optimum conditions of therapeutic interaction.

Killian and Clark (1996) observe that most nurses have to work out for themselves, the right balance between their custodial and more clinical role. Open discussion of dilemmas is rare, e.g. "what it means to lock up in seclusion a person with whom they have established a close relationship, often over a period of years."

These observations seem to provide one of the first realistic accounts of the real difficulties forensic nurses experience in their work. That includes role conflict which is an inherent part of their work and which has to be managed. Traditionally though, there has been little precedent for guidance. Kitchener *et al.* (1992) had already identified that conflict and ambiguity associated with forensic nurses' therapeutic and controlling roles were common problems. Nursing staff unable to negotiate the psychodynamic agenda, are likely to avoid confronting necessarily complex psychological processes which are in any event often unpalatable. Tension, between traditional nursing interventions; with their roots in caring for less able individuals during periods in their lives when they are unable to fulfil these tasks for themselves due to illness or disability, and the pathological dynamics which are at play when long stay but largely able bodied individuals, who may have no adaptive framework through which to process care and nurturing interventions, must be most apparent in forensic services.

Conclusions

Nursing in secure environments requires a concentration of staff with specific expertise who have considerable continuing professional development needs and supervision requirements. Nurses are key professionals in these environments and have responsibility for providing nursing interventions and for maintaining much of the security framework and processes within which these interventions take place. Key issues in secure environments relate to the standards for; the preparation of nurses to work in these areas, the development of occupational and professional competence, the difficulty of developing professional practice in 'closed' institutions and the complexity of interpersonal and professional relationships with patients.

Evidence from a wide range of sources on policy and practice in secure hospital settings was reviewed to provide a comprehensive overview of the historical context of secure mental health care; contemporary arrangements for care in these settings; the demands imposed by the current epidemiology of relevant disorders, and a range of service development issues.

The following issues were identified:

- The problems of caring for those deemed dangerously mentally ill is and is likely to remain a long-standing public policy problem.

- Beds in secure care for mentally disordered offenders have increased significantly in England over the last 10 years. Secure provision and consequently nursing in secure care is likely to be a significant and enduring feature of provision for these groups in the future.

- Problems in secure mental care are exacerbated by lack of through put and step down to general psychiatric services.

- A number of reports have recommended greater variety and range of secure provision with higher levels of community input but with little actual change in service provision being effected.

- The in-patient population is largely composed of people with serious and enduring mental illness: in-patients have higher levels of disadvantage, social exclusion, homelessness, and a much broader and more complex set of needs than they did in the past. The number of patients who have problems both with substance abuse dependence and a mental illness has risen steeply. Patients with a dual diagnosis place great demands on the clinical skills of nurses, who are often not trained to provide the complexity of care required.

- The lack of understanding and knowledge about race and culture, institutional racism, euro-centric assumptions, and the racist attitudes of some of those involved in the various services is a common theme from the literature.

- Professional education, and research, should take account of issues of race and culture and that all agencies should identify staff training needs and establish programmes to address these concerns.

- People with a Learning Disability are reducing in number in higher levels of secure care.

- Amongst current admissions, the largest single groups are those with a history of violence against the person. Patients convicted or prosecuted for sexual offences have increased 3 fold in the last 10 years.

- Health Secure environments continue to care for a predominantly young population.

- It is difficult for professionals to distinguish between the range of clinical problems and treatment needs of individuals with different diagnoses and different levels of security.

- Though developing at a different pace, strategic developments for care of those requiring secure care are taking place in the same direction across the UK.

- Although beyond the scope of this study some evidence appears to suggest that mental health nurses in general mental health services are ill equipped to deal with rehabilitation and ongoing treatment of those passing down through the system.

- There is a need to further develop the theoretical and practice base of nursing in relation to the range of psychopathologies of forensic patients.

- Nurses working in secure environments face significant and enduring role conflict in attempting to reconcile their responsibilities for therapeutic care and maintaining security, which can be in conflict. This principally stems from the ambiguity of working with clients who are simultaneously patients and prisoners/detainees.

- Patients in these populations have extremely complex health, social, psychological and forensic backgrounds all of which impose complex demands on their nursing care on a day to day basis.

2.2 The Development of Health Care in Prisons

Pegram (1997) provides a comprehensive background to the development of the nursing role within the Prison Services. "Towards the end of the nineteenth century the Gladstone Report of 1895 argued that the Prison system should be more flexible and discriminating, capable of both responding to the needs of individual prisoners and of helping to make prisoners better men and women when they left prison. As the different needs of prisoners were recognised so specialists from outside were introduced into prisons, the earliest of these in the nineteenth century being the doctor who was assisted by prison officers, called hospital officers, more recently named health care officers." (Pegram 1997)

The emphasis on reformation in the Prison Services across the UK, over the first half of the twentieth century, found expression in the placing of the treatment objective as, "the purpose of the training and treatment of convicted prisoners shall be to encourage and assist them to lead a good and useful life" (Prison Rules Act 1964). Treatment in this context refers to "good treatment" or "inhuman treatment" which is consistent with the long-standing moral purpose of imprisonment i.e. reform. Walker(1968) refers to the Gladstone Committee of 1895, which stated that "prison treatment should be effectively designed to maintain, stimulate, or awaken the higher susceptibilities of prisoners and turn them out of prison better men and women, both physically and morally, than when they came in". Walker notes that this "has been adopted as an article of faith by the prison administration of today".

From the mid 1960's the confidence in the treatment objective of prisons had appeared to wane, partly because research findings about the effectiveness of treatment regimes in checking recidivism were discouraging (The May Committee 1977), and partly because of crises in prisons which diverted resources away from the treatment objective. This gave rise to emphasis on "humane containment" based on the concept that prisoners are committed to prisons as a punishment, not for punishment (The May Committee 1977). A major riot at HMP Manchester in 1990 provoked copycat disturbances throughout the prison system. The Government commissioned a report into the prison disturbances (The Woolf Report 1991) and following its publication a statement of purpose was issued stating "Her Majesty's Prison Services serves the public by keeping in custody those committed by the courts. Our duty is to look after them with humanity and help them lead law-abiding and useful lives in custody and after release".

In response to a report on the Management of the Prison Services (Lygo 1991), the Prison Service, in England and Wales, became an "Executive Agency" on 1 April 1993, this meant that Government ministers while still remaining ultimately responsible to Parliament for the Prison Service's operations, were to be less involved in the day to day running of the service. In Scotland a similar process resulted in the Scottish Prison Service (SPS) also becoming an executive agency and Northern Ireland's Prison Service became an agency in 1995.

Within the United Kingdom there are three Prison Services, England and Wales, Scotland and Northern Ireland. These services have developed to reflect the needs of the populations, but also many of the developments have been in parallel with the other countries; health care services within Prisons being one example. In 1993 the Scottish Prison Service

C   Prisoners who cannot be trusted in open conditions but who do not have the ability or resources to make determined effort to escape

D   Prisoners who can be reasonably trusted to serve their sentences in open conditions

Categories B, C and D are only for adult convicted men. Unconvicted prisoners, unless they are category A, will not be categorised, but are usually treated as category B. Women and Young Offenders, if they are not classed as category A, will only be classed as suitable for "open" or "closed" prisons. If a prisoner has a long sentence, his or her category may be changed from time to time to a lower one. Alternatively, if they try to escape or if the prison discovers information that a prisoner is dangerous, it may be changed to a higher one. (Prison Libraries Group 1998). In Northern Ireland, categorisation is either, high, medium, low or remand

Type of Facility	Total	Male	Female	Mixed
Closed Training Prison	48	43	4	1
Open Training Prison	12	9	3	
Local Prison	55	41	5	5
Dispersal Prison	10	9		1
Young Offenders Institution	31	31		
Immigration Detention Centre	1	1		
Total	157			

Table 2.2.1. Types of Prison Facilities in England and Wales, Scotland and Northern Ireland

The Prison Population

The size of the prison population has historically depended upon the attitudes of the Government in power and society at large. The prison population in England and Wales has risen steadily over the past four decades to 61,100 in 1997, and in the same year, in Scotland there were 6,084 inmates, the average for 1998 was 6,026. In Northern Ireland the 1997 figure was 1,611, but this is reducing, in 1998 the average prison population was 1,494 and in 1999 it is 1,306

	Men	Women	Young Offenders (Male and Female)
England and Wales	47,610	2,680	10,810
Scotland	5,132	165	787
Northern Ireland	1,322	30	237

Table 2.2.2 Average Prison Population 1997

Ethnic Minorities within the Prison Population

The representation of ethnic minorities within the prison populations varies across the three services. In Scotland and Northern Ireland the prison population of ethnic minorities reflects the general population, but in England and Wales there is a significant variance.

In 1997, in Scottish prisons there were 79 non-whites (1.3%), 78 were male, imprisoned, this is a similar proportion to that of ethnic minorities in the Scottish population as a whole (Scottish Office 1998). Northern Ireland does not keep specific statistics on ethnic minorities, but the Press Office of the Northern Ireland Prison Service have stated that the small numbers of ethnic minority prisoners is a reflection of the general population (Northern Ireland Office 1999).

In England and Wales, in the same period, 10,827 (18%) of males and 2,672 (24%) of females were non-white, with black males (12%) and black females (19%) being the highest proportions. This is an over representation as black males make up only 1% and black females 2% of the general population in England and Wales (Home Office 1998).

Nature of the Client Group

The *Future Organisation of Prison Health Care* (HM Prison Service and NHS Executive 1999) reports that during the period April 1996 to March 1997 staff providing health care in prisons in England and Wales handled over 2 million consultations with inmates. About two thirds of these involved contact with a nurse or health care officers, 27% with prison doctors and about 9% with NHS specialists visiting prisons (HM Prison Service and NHS Executive 1999). Although data available from individual prisons suggests that this figure may be an underestimation of the actual workload on nurses working in prisons.

The prison populations are made up disproportionately of men who drink and smoke heavily, have more active health problems than the population at large, and show evidence of self-neglect. Amongst the older group of inmates there are a large number of alcoholics serving short sentences for drink related offences. The men in prison are under abnormal amounts of stress and have violent tendencies (Social Services Committee 1985). Other research has shown that prisoners suffer from high levels of mental disorder, drug misuse and general poor health (Birmingham *et al.* 1996; Brooke *et al.* 1996; Bellis *et al.* 1997; Mason *et al.* 1997). Martin (1989) in his anecdotal article concerning prison medicine mentions that the patients/prisoners are largely from social classes IV and V. He continues that there is a high incidence of mental illness and psychopathy and discusses a survey conducted at Bedford prison which found that as a group, prisoners tend to neglect their health and have a high alcohol intake.(Walsh 1998) This view is supported by the data collected during the 1997 survey *Psychiatric morbidity among prisoners in England and Wales* (Office for National Statistics 1997)

The Prison Service in Scotland reports that it deals both with prisoners whose mental disorder may be appropriate for medical intervention and those whose disturbed behaviour is not the result of mental disorder as defined earlier (see section 2.1). While the number of prisoners with psychotic illness who might be accepted for transfer to hospital is quite small, research suggests that the rate of psychological disturbance in Scottish prisons could be at least twice that in the general population and perhaps even higher among female prisoners. (Scottish Office 1998)

Some 10% of the prison population report sick each day (Wool 1993), a rate some eight times higher than the attendance rate of the general population at their general practitioners. Due to the fact that 95% of the prison population are under 50 years of age, it has been suggested that a substantial proportion of prisoners reporting sick has little to do with health or sickness, but is more likely to be the result of "medicalisation" of more general problems such as the inability of some vulnerable prisoners to cope with prison life (Acheson 1993). Unlike the general public the prison population has no access to household remedies that would normally be purchased over the counter at local pharmacies. Prisoners are often suspected of exaggerating symptoms or manipulating in order to get drugs or medicines that their condition did not merit. (Walsh 1998)

Rodriguez (1994) mentions that health problems inside prisons are similar to those outside but that they are in a higher proportion than would be expected in people of the same age group in the community. The following table highlights the extent of some of the health problems for prisoners in England and Wales that are dealt with by health care workers in prison:

Illness 1 Condition	Total Number of Inmates (1996/7)
Self Harm Incidents	5,360
Diabetics	476
Asthmatics	3,185
Known HIV positive inmates	105
Inmates receiving treatment for mental health problems	1,887
Notifiable drug addicts	13,181
Non notifiable drug addicts	8,839

Table 2.2.3 Health care issues in prison
(Source: Table compiled from Longfield 1998)

The mental health care of prisoners requires a significant input from heath care staff and presents nurses with a number of ethical issues. For example, under the Mental Health Act (1983) prison hospitals are classified as "places of safety" and as such medication and treatment are voluntary and not compulsory, nurses are therefore, under the Mental Health Act, unable to treat a violent patient against his/her will. This contrasts sharply with the situation in psychiatric hospitals where under section 62 of the Mental Health Act (1983), urgent treatment may be given without the patient's consent under specified conditions. Therefore, since health care staff working in the Prison Services have no recourse to the use of medication in these circumstances to treat violent clients, they are often left with only one option, that is the use of physical restraints. (Pegram 1997)

While the figures for reported assaults on nurses working in the NHS appear high, health care staff in prisons, in England and Wales have a 1 in 4 chance of being assaulted each year (HM Prison Service 1993). That is 18 times more likely than nurses working in the NHS and almost 4,000 times more likely than members of the general public. It must also be borne in mind that the figures for reported assaults on staff in prisons do not reflect the true levels of violence, and these figures relate to all prison health care staff, not just nurses.

The Provision of Health Care within Prisons

Within the public Prison Services the Governor is primarily responsible for the prison health care services. As part of the general thrust of devolution of management responsibility that the service has seen in the last few years, Governors are not obliged to follow any one particular model. The way in which Health Centres are organised therefore vary both in management, staffing mix and number. The costs for health care provided within the prison are borne against prison budgets. In contractually managed prisons health care is provided against a specification that forms part of the contract between the Prison Services and the Contractor.

The delivery of health care within HM Prisons in the UK falls primarily on health care staff who fall into one of the following categories: prison service nurses; health care officers with nursing qualifications; and health care officers without nursing and qualifications; contracted in services such as midwifery or Community Psychiatric Nursing Services.

The Future Organisation of Prison Health Care report (HM Prison and NHS Executive 1999) indicates that in England and Wales "Over the last few years Registered Nurses have been recruited but without a meaningful assessment of the knowledge and skills required. Their particular competencies have not often been utilised to the full." The document contained an aspiration that "in future, all nursing care" would be "under the supervision of a first level registered nurse". In England and Wales many health care managers and team leader posts, however, continue to be held by Senior and Principal Health Care Officers or Governor grades without nursing registration. In March 1998, 11 Prisons reported having no registered nurses in clinical or supervisory posts.

The situation in Scotland and Northern Ireland is different, as can be seen from the following table. Non-nurse qualified Health Care Officers are a feature of health care provision in England and Wales and Northern Ireland, whereas Scotland now has a full complement of registered nurses.

	England & Wales		Scotland		Northern Ireland	
Prison Service Nurses	879	53.2%	161	100%	18	22%
Health Care Officers (nurse qualified)	288	17.4%	NIL	NIL	12	15%
Health Care Officers (non-nurse qualified)	486	29.4%	NIL	NIL	52	63%

Table 2.2.4 Profile Of Health Care Staff At March 1999

(Source - HM Prison Service, England and Wales, Scottish Prison Service, Northern Ireland)

Nurse qualified Health Care Officers have a dual clinical and custodial role, the delivery of nursing care and the full duties of a prison officer, while Prison Services nurses' role is exclusively clinical.

Attempts have been made to define the health care roles within the Prison Services. The role of the nurse or the health care officer is defined in England and Wales by Home Office Standing Order 13 (Health Care) as:

- Carrying out basic nursing care and such specialist nursing care as within their competence.
- Observing patients in their charge and alerting a Medical Officer to any matters relating to the health or treatment of a patient which are considered to warrant medical attention.
- Keeping accurate records of medicine administered and other significant nursing duties undertaken, as required by the Managing Medical Officer.
- Advising Medical Officers on the statutory provisions, Standing Orders and Headquarters Instructions and general guidance relevant to the performance of their duties generally or the procedure in a particular case. (Home Office 1991)

Dr Rosemary J. Wool, the Director of Health Care Services for Prisoners expanded upon this definition, in a policy statement issued on 16 October 1992. This document states that: "...the experience, skills and interests of individual members of the nursing staff will make it necessary for management to determine the appropriate skill mix with advice from the Directorate of Health Care. The role of nursing staff will be extended and enhanced to include services such as counselling and health education. The greater emphasis in future on preventative medicine, health education and health promotion which can be expected to evolve from the establishment of the Health Care Service for Prisoners and will provide further opportunities for such work making the job of nursing staff more satisfying and rewarding. There are advantages in nursing grades gravitating between the National Health Service and the Nursing Service for Prisoners, it is one valuable means of refreshing prison nursing and keeping the Service in tune with the ethos and methods of the National Health Service". (Wool 1992)

Therapy versus Security

Doctors and nursing staff within the Health Care service for prisoners work in a unique environment and they have the problem of being viewed by their clientele as being a source of treatment, comfort and advice but at the same time as being part of the system that has deprived them of their liberty. This results in many prisoners mistrusting or refusing to use the facilities available to promote their health. (Walsh 1998)

The following table, cited by Walsh (1998), illustrates the differences in what Stevens (1993) terms folkways and morals between prison and health care. These comparisons appear to reflect not only the publics' perception of services provided in these settings, but also the stereotyping by the media. Within the services visited there were occasions when these views were expressed by nurses themselves, either as a rationale for the way in which they deliver nursing care, or as an issue that they felt needed addressing to enable them to deliver appropriate care to individuals irrespective of the setting in which they were employed.

Element	Health Care	Prison
Folkways	Comfort measures	Keys & Cells
	Touch	No touching
	Belief in patients	Disbelief of inmates
	Uniforms	Uniforms
	Frequently alone	Never alone - security risk
Morals	Trust / respect	No trust
	Softness / Acceptance	Tough attitude
	Kindness is expected by providers	Kindness leads to a "set up" and personnel will be taken advantage of

Table 2.2.5 The differences in folkways and morals between prison and health care

An efficiency scrutiny of the Prison Medical Service, examining the effectiveness and value for money of the Prison Service's arrangements for providing medical services for prisoners commented that "Hospital Officers (renamed Health Care Officers) combined the roles of discipline and health care. These are difficult roles to combine. Some hospital officers clearly had a very caring attitude but in others the discipline role had almost completely subjugated the care role" (Scrutiny Team 1990). The Scrutiny Team also commented that "nurses would bring with them an image and attitude towards care which would enhance health care work". While this report did not directly examine the subject of role conflict for prison health care staff, it did acknowledge that a conflict of roles exists. This creates an inordinate role conflict for these staff who are required to fuse these two dimensions together. This role conflict is further confused by the UKCC Code of Professional Conduct (1998), in the introductory statements registered nurses are asked to: "a) safeguard and promote the interests of individual patients and clients; and b) serve the interests of society". At times, within a secure environment, these two objectives conflict. (Walsh 1998)

This security/therapy tension often results in patient scepticism towards the health care staff's actions and motives. This mistrust can work in the opposite direction, when working with clients who have already shown a disregard for the accepted rules of society and have perhaps displayed a propensity for violence and dangerousness, the health care staff working in the prison environment must exercise a benign scepticism. That is to say that an awareness exists that some patients may attempt to exploit certain situations in order to undermine the integrity of security procedures to gain some personal advantage. (Walsh 1998)

It is clear from the discussions with participants and from the literature, including Walsh 1998, Pegram 1997 and Wilmott 1997, that health care staff working in the Health Care Service for Prisoners find the conflict of interests difficult. Walsh(1998) suggests that this is most likely because, as individuals, they are all orientated either more emphatically towards therapeutic interventions or uncompromisingly towards custodial considerations. Their stance on these issues may derive from the differing social and political values that they hold as members of a broad culture. Health care staff reflect every shade on the opinion of the management of this client group. Some may be indifferent towards the residents for whom they are responsible while the knowledge of their patients past actions and the constant threat of potential violence may disturb others. One study (Phillips 1983) on the attitudes of Canadian nurses working in secure environments revealed that 17% of respondents viewed their client group as criminals rather than patients, there have been no studies of this type undertaken in the UK which either refute or support this statement.

Although there is a regular debate about "security versus therapy" nurses working in these settings have to integrate aspects of both in order to develop care programmes that meet the individuals needs as well as maintaining security. Whilst it must be acknowledged that the confinement of a prisoner in a secure environment is primarily in the interest of the public rather than the individual, best practice today should attempt to work from the belief that security is not necessarily at odds with treatment goals and is best incorporated where possible into care plans.

Competing Cultures?

In a discussion paper issued by Her Majesty's Inspectorate of Prisons for England and Wales, it was stated that "There should be greater clarification of differences between the responsibilities of medical staff and the day to day workings of the establishment. At present a patient, presenting him or herself for medical attention, is faced by nursing staff with a variety of uniforms, grades and qualifications within the same establishment. Some are in Prison Officer uniform, with or without a nursing qualification. Others are in different uniforms. probably with nursing qualifications." (HM Inspectorate of Prisons 1996). In Northern Ireland this issue has been resolved through the issue of tunic and trousers to all health care staff irrespective of their discipline.

There is pressure on prison health centres with inpatient facilities to operate at 100% occupancy resulting in the non-clinical use of health care accommodation. *The Future Organisation of Prison Health Care* report (HM Prison Service 1999) identifies statutory duties and prison rules are not geared for effective delivery of primary care. They do not recognise the responsibilities of each healthcare team member and lead to inappropriate use of time. It went on to report that "We were also struck by the frequent use of prison healthcare centres to manage prisoners who failed to cope on the prison wings and for whom social support would be more appropriate than medical care". (HM Prison Service and NHS Executive 1999)

Walsh (1999) cites a report on work in Canada where Droes (1994) reports that "In discussing the special world where the nursing work occurs, the structural conditions of the correctional setting hold consequences for nursing care to inmates. Structural conditions are elaborated further in three areas - a) the ever present security measures, b) inadequate facilities, equipment and supplies and c) insufficient staffing." Droes highlighted the ever-present security measures as the most profound factor in the delivery of nursing care.

The interactions between various individuals and groups within the correctional setting hold consequences for nursing practice. (Droes 1994) This study discovered that "custody's toleration of healthcare was the most notable in the interactions between custody staff and health care staff" (Droes 1994). Droes continued to describe a continuum of toleration of health care by custody staff. At one end of the continuum, contentious toleration of health care occurred where "custody staff accepted inmate health care grudgingly and viewed it as a distraction and interference with the performance of their own work". At the other end of this continuum, this is considered toleration which "denoted situations in which custody staff evaluated health care as not only benefiting inmates but also assisting in the performance of their own work". (Droes 1994)

This study drew two main conclusions: Firstly that custody staff exert significant influence on the correctional health care environment and secondly that nurses working in the correctional environment with increased levels of education and experience in public health are prepared to provide a broader scope of health care to inmates. Therefore the most favourable conditions for health care delivery in prisons occurred when there was considered toleration by correctional officers and an expanded conception of nursing by nurses.

The Future Organisation of Prison Health Care report adds to this view. They report that "Prisons where nurses had been empowered as organisational managers and clinical leaders appeared to have more consistent and professional delivery of care. However, the potential to use nurses most cost effectively has in many instances been missed due to inflexible employment practices and inexperience in managing nurses' terms and conditions of employment. Some nursing staff commented that they were often required to perform tasks inappropriate to their skills resulting in less then optimum use of their abilities and hence a less efficient service. Some staff commented that they were not able to realise their full potential. (HM Prison Service and NHS Executive 1999)

Nurses in the Gulotta study (1987) felt that the goals of the correctional administration and the nursing service were in opposition. This implies that the goals of security and nursing are in conflict with one another leading to the care versus custody dilemma. Although changes have taken place, particularly in Scotland, this view is again expressed in the Future Organisation of Prison Health Care, one of the action points identified is to separate the care and custody functions.

The following extract from *Future Organisation of Prison Health Care* outlines a potential way forward for prison nursing:

"The role of nurses in prisons needs to be based on a more flexible and effective model of nurse competencies, focusing on the impact that nurses can make on health promotion and illness prevention. Psychiatric nurses with experience of forensic settings, risk management, the management of violence and skills in therapeutic approaches such as cognitive therapy would greatly improve the care of mentally disordered offenders."

"It is generally accepted that:

- There is a national shortage of trained nurses (in England) and the extent to which the Prison Services are successful in recruiting nurses depends on the Service's image and the perception that the nursing profession has on the opportunities and career structure that is offered.
- The custodial setting is unlikely to prove attractive to many, and the current isolated nature of prison health care must be regarded as a significant disincentive. Barriers to effective recruitment and retention need to be removed." (HM Prison Service and NHS Executive 1999)

Given the wide variation in size and type of prison establishments it would be difficult to be precise about the model of nursing services. However, nursing leadership needs to be supported overtly by governors and other managers. In particular nurses must be enabled to practice within their ethical framework, the Code of Professional Conduct. A new national strategy for nursing in the NHS is currently being prepared following widespread consultation. It is essential that nursing in prisons reflects the standards the NHS is striving to achieve. The national strategy is expected to enhance and strengthen the contribution of nurses within a multi-professional, multi-agency approach.

Underpinned by the principle of equivalence, it was the view of *the Future Organisation of Prison Health Care* Working Group that healthcare of a nursing nature should be led by qualified nurses. We see this as supportive of the general move towards separating custodial and nursing functions. We recognise that this will have a significant impact on the existing Health Care Officers. Those Health Care Officers who satisfy selection criteria should be enabled to undertake nurse training in the light of assessed health needs and skill shortages. For those who do not wish or are unable to acquire nursing qualifications we would see appropriate therapeutic roles in the context of developed regimes for dealing with prisoners with mental disorder, and supporting initiatives to provide community mental health support and social care in prisons. In the multidisciplinary healthcare team, health care officers have a key role to play." (HM Prison Service and NHS Executive 1999)

Conclusions

Evidence from a wide range of sources on policy and practice in prison health care settings was reviewed to provide a comprehensive overview of the historical context of prison health care; contemporary arrangements for care in these settings; the demands imposed by the current epidemiology of relevant disorders, and a range of service development issues. The problems facing nurses working in a prison environment are summed up by a health care co-ordinator quoted by Day (1983) who states

"The clients with whom we deal are complex individuals. Some are manipulators and or malingerers. Some are genuine. Some are drug addicts and many have alcohol problems. Some use the system, others utilise it. They are men, women and transsexuals. Some are retarded, some psychotic, some depressed, some "normal", and they present a variety of physical conditions including diabetes, heart problems, multiple sclerosis, arthritis and even pregnancy. On the whole, the nurse patient relationship is congenial, but this does not alter the fact that these individuals lead a life much different from our own and have a value system that may not correspond to ours".

The following issues were identified:

- There is a deliberate, specific policy in each of the three Prison Services to use registered nurses as one of the key components of care for prisoners.

- In all 3 Prison Services (England and Wales, Scotland and Northern Ireland) there has been a move to recognise prisoners rights to appropriate health care and to accept its importance from a humane and rehabilitative perspective.

- Recruitment and retention of nurses is an issue that needs to be addressed in order to maintain an effective and efficient nursing workforce

- Historically, health care in the prison has been developed within the service as an element of the regime rather than being developed as part of the NHS.

- Difference in local management arrangements and priorities within the Prison Services, have on occasions made the implementation of service wide standards of health care extremely difficult.

- Patients' rights and access to health care have been influenced by prisoners' legal action rather than based on health need.

- The range of health needs of prisoners is extremely diverse and includes severe mental illness, personality disorder, poor physical health, drug and alcohol dependency, trauma, primary care and health promotion.

- Historical personnel and occupational arrangements within the Prison Services, especially in England, have meant that the specific role and contribution of nurses has been unclear and confused with the custodial role of prison officers.

3.0 Method of data collection used in the scoping exercise

Locations and Sampling

The project brief required a comprehensive overview of nursing in secure environments across the UK both within hospitals and the Prison Services. The sampling frame had to take account of the lack of aggregated information about locations where secure provision is available and the numbers of nurses employed. The methods used needed to be realistic about what was feasible within the time-scale and the number of stakeholders and secure environments the study needed to embrace.

In studying the practice environments the key difficulty appears that the systems of criminal justice and health services have little in common in relation to their structure and organisation, and the distribution of nurses within them is quite different.

This can best be exemplified by a comparison of nursing in prisons and nursing in High Secure Hospitals. There are currently 1359 nurses employed in the 3 prison nursing services in 157 establishments. To establish as clear a picture as possible a total survey was attempted. The situation in the high security forensic psychiatric services gives a totally different sampling problem, since a similar number of nurses is concentrated in a very small number of establishments. There are 3 hospitals covering England and Wales, and 1 in Scotland, with similar admission criteria, all offering twenty-four-hour in-patient psychiatric care. They employ in the region of 2,000 qualified nurses. Clearly a randomised sample of this population would be feasible and a suggested 20 % of each nursing clinical grade (C to I) was proposed for the staff questionnaire.

In the medium and low security settings where work to date has identified 38 medium secure units and 96 Low secure units (Rampton Hospital Forensic Directory and personal inquiry at NHSE Regional Offices). A sample of 8 medium and 16 low secure units was randomly selected from the database of services identified. Although no questionnaires were distributed to nurses in the health sector in Northern Ireland, nurses from the Prison Services and hospitals participated in the focus groups and through the audit process, and questionnaires were completed by nurses in the Northern Ireland Prison Service.

Data Analysis

As this study is descriptive in its approach, quantitative and qualitative information was collected from the respondents in order to discover, describe and compare themes. Data analysis included a mixture of both quantitative and qualitative processes and included the following:

1. Quantitative analysis of data emerging from the questionnaires and audit document by the use of descriptive statistical techniques in the form of graphic presentations and frequency tables;

2. Qualitative descriptions of data emerging from the questionnaire, focus groups and focus interviews;

3. Qualitative descriptions of comparisons made between questionnaire, audit, focus group and focused interviews and literature review findings.

Methodology

The breadth of the study's objectives indicated that no single research method would be sufficient to generate the depth and richness of data required. It was proposed that data be obtained using a range of research methods.

The main methods were:

- Literature search
- Focus groups
- Interviews
- Questionnaires
- Audits and observation

Literature search

An exploratory review of the international literature relating to secure health and prison care. This encompassed the main electronic sources, including:-

ASSIA
Caredata
Cinahl
Medline/Psychlit
RCN Nurse ROM

The literature search resulted in the production of a bibliography spanning over 680 references from 147 different periodicals, journals and books spanning 18 years of publications including 425 authors. These appear in the bibliography appended to the report. (Appendix 6.8)

An exploratory review of the literature relating to secure nursing and forensic care was undertaken. This encompassed the main electronic sources of medical, nursing and social sciences literature. In addition, hand searching of key journals and examination of unpublished 'grey literature', together with Internet searches, was carried out to enhance the validity of the literature review.

Focus groups

A total of 22 Focus Groups were conducted with over 250 participants. The Focus Groups were held with both nurses working in prisons and hospital nurses across the four UK countries to ensure that a representative sample was obtained. (See Appendices 3 and 4 for organisations represented and venues where focus groups were held)

Focus groups are a form of group interview that capitalises on communication between research participants in order to generate data. The method is especially appropriate when working with disempowered groups, who are often reluctant to give negative feedback, or who may feel that any problems they encounter result from their own inadequacies; and are an effective technique for exploring staff attitudes and needs.

The groups were guided through the objectives, and appropriate points recorded in note form. The focus groups were held at locations throughout the UK, and were semi-structured in approach. A focus group plan was developed to ensure consistency of approach and that all the key areas are covered in the sessions, together with a field note reporting form based on work by Krueger (1994). It was decided at an early stage to run separate criminal justice and health service groups as sector specific issues might prevent constructive discussion.

The data generated was codified and used to contribute to the list of issues identified and in the development of the three questionnaires.

Interviews

A series of 34 interviews either face to face or by telephone, were carried out, focusing on a specific purposive sub-sample. This method has been defined as "a type of non- probability sampling in which the researcher selects subjects for the study on the basis of personal judgement about which ones will be most representative or productive" (Polit and Hungler 1989). This interview technique was used to ensure that all relevant subject areas were covered, including those defined by respondents.

Interviews were conducted with identified individuals who it was felt had a significant contribution to make to the objectives of the scoping exercise. This included the acknowledged experts in the field, senior managers and opinion formers, researchers, educationalists and clinical staff (Polit and Hungler 1989). (Appendix 2 contains information on individuals interviewed during this scoping exercise)

These interviews were used to confirm some of the emerging information from the focus groups and generate new information from the interviewee's own experiences and observations. A semi-structured interview schedule was developed together with a field note reporting form (based on Krueger 1994). Contemporaneous notes of the individual interviews were subjected to codifying for analysis purposes and for formulating the questionnaires.

Questionnaires

From the outset questionnaires were identified as one of the core research instruments to gather data in response to the seven key questions set for the secure environments project. This decision to use questionnaires was based on the need to gather data from as wide a range of participants as possible given the time scales and UK wide dimension.

Three questionnaires were developed during the exercise, these being:

- The Educational Questionnaire was intended to involve a total sample of Universities in the UK which offered Mental Health and Learning Disabilities programmes at pre and post registration. From the 65 questionnaires distributed 38 (58%) responses were received.

- The Organisational Questionnaire was also intended to involve a total sample of Prisons and those Hospitals that provided secure care. Questionnaires were circulated to 157 Prisons and 138 high, medium and low secure hospitals. The returns were 61 (39%) from prisons and 54 (39%) from hospitals.

- The Staff Questionnaire was sent to nurses in both sectors

   It was intended as

   - A total survey of all nurses working in Prisons. 1359 questionnaires were circulated to nurses working in prison with 435 responses (31.5%).
   - A stratified (by grade) random sample (20%) in two of the high secure hospitals; this attracted 70 responses (43%)
   - A randomised sample of all staff in 8 medium secure units; with 143 (31%) responses
   - A randomised sample involving staff from 16 low security units: 66 (30%) responses were received.

A total of 714 responses have been analysed within the report.

Rationale

The starting point for questionnaire development was therefore the key objectives themselves; and initially a single questionnaire was developed. It became apparent that different types of information, from different sources, were required and that it would be beneficial to design separate questionnaires; one to be completed by a knowledgeable individual on behalf of the employing organisation (the organisational questionnaire) and one to be completed by individual nurses (the staff questionnaire). It was also considered of value to survey the program leaders for Mental Health and Learning Disability pre-registration and post- registration nursing programmes, in order to examine the issue of preparation of nurses for working in secure environments (the educational preparation questionnaire).

The final questionnaires incorporated issues raised through the focus group and focus interview processes and were used to test out ideas and theories generated from these earlier data gathering methods.

Once the questionnaires were finalised a pilot study was conducted with a number of individuals within the health sector and the Prison Services to ascertain if the questions were understandable; if individuals were likely to make mistakes; and how long they would take to complete (Waterman 1998).

In an attempt to increase the response rate the potential respondents received: a short letter stating the study aims; how the person was chosen; reassurance that data would be treated confidentially (and what that meant); details of the organisation carrying out the study; and obvious personal relevance of the topic area to the respondent.

Although the % rate of responses to the staff questionnaire were relatively low, the total of 714 returns provides sufficient data from which to develop our conclusions and recommendations.

Audit and Observation

18 audit and observation visits were made to hospitals and prisons. (The results from the audit are shown in Appendix 6)

As well as receiving feedback from individuals providing and receiving services, it was important to reach a judgement as to whether current guidelines on good practice are in use within the work environments, not least the UKCC guidelines themselves. The researchers observed and measured both availability and utilisation of these guidelines against agreed standards in the form of a checklist. A small number of audits were undertaken at all levels of security within the health care sector and at levels 1-3 of health care centres within the Prison Services.

The audit tool comprised of a checklist against which to measure service delivery in practice. This required an examination of records and record keeping, policies and procedures in the clinical setting and looked for the physical evidence to support assertions. This was undoubtedly the most contentious method used; however, if a true picture of direct nursing practice was to be gained then it was essential that this method be utilised. (Dale 1990)

Validity and Reliability Studies

According to Polit and Hungler (1993) "an instrument can be said to be reliable if its measures accurately reflect the true measures of the attribute under investigation". The research instruments were designed to collect information that is essentially qualitative in nature therefore the responses could not be treated as stable. Opinions and views may change over a period of time following the influences of new information received. Therefore, although the data received was quantified, where possible, for ease of analysis, reliability tests for use on quantitative data were not used.

Polit and Hungler (1993) define validity as "the degree to which an instrument measures what it is supposed to be measuring". There are a number of processes involved in establishing the validity of an instrument but it has to be accepted that this is an extremely difficult thing to achieve with a new instrument that is designed specifically for use in a study. The researchers endeavoured to establish fact and content validity by submitting the questionnaire to a small panel of subject experts and experienced researchers. This panel was asked to constructively criticise the instruments; and their suggestions were included in the finalised research instruments.

4.0 Key Issues for the Scoping Exercise

The following section provides an analysis of the literature and responses from the focus groups, focused interviews, questionnaires and audits in relation to the seven key issues, which are

4.1 Describe the competencies required of nurses working in secure environments

4.2 Are nurses interventions in secure environments evidence based?

4.3 Review current activity in the development of practice standards in secure environments, particularly with reference to specific client groups

4.4 How effective is the preparation currently given to nurses working in secure environments?

4.5 Identify issues faced in working with a client group who may compromise therapeutic nurse patient relationships, particularly with reference to personality disordered patients

4.6 Identify the extent to which existing Council policies are utilised and inform practice within secure environments

4.7 Identify practice issues relevant to the physical health needs of these populations; care of women (including care of pregnant women); care of people from different cultural backgrounds

4.1 Describe the competencies required of nurses working in secure environments

The issue of competence to practice is one that has been debated in nursing for a number of years. The main issues "Fitness for Practice", "Fitness for Purpose" and "Fitness for Award" (UKCC 1999), are particularly relevant to the preparation and development of nurses who work in secure environments.

The UKCC (1997) have identified that "Competence based approaches to vocational and professional development have been increasingly advocated by UK Governments and employers. Nurse education must reflect these needs. Higher Education institutions offer a wide range of National Board validated specialist practitioner courses but there does not appear to be a common understanding of competence to practice across providers nor consensus on appropriate methods of assessing that competence".

Competence models can come in a number of forms:

- "what people should be like"- models based on personal characteristics or an individuals behaviour
- "what people need to possess"- models based on acquiring knowledge, understanding and skills
- "what people need to achieve in the workplace"- models based on outcomes and standards including underpinning knowledge and skills (Mitchell 1998)

There are a significant number of definitions and types of competence described in the nursing and wider professional literature. (WHO 1988, Hogston 1993, UKCC 1989, Mansfield and Mitchell 1996)

In attempting to identify the competencies required of nurses working in a secure environment the "Job Competence Model" described by Mansfield and Matthews (1985) provided a framework for development. This model suggests that work roles have four interrelated components, all of which are present in all activity. The components are described as: *technical expectations* - achieving the expectations of the work role which characterise the occupation; *managing contingencies* - recognising and resolving potential and actual breakdowns in processes and procedures, including coping with emergencies; *managing different work activities* - achieving balance and co-ordinating a number of different and potentially conflicting activities to lead to the successful conclusion of aims and goals; and *managing the interface with the work environment* - achieving the expectations which arise from natural constraints, the quality measures which are applied, the nature of work organisation and the nature of working relationships.

Many of the competencies described in professional publications fall into one or more of the categories described in the Job Competence Model. Together the competencies needed to undertake a given role in forensic nursing should prepare practitioners who are fit for purpose and fit to practice. Competencies are needed to provide a recognition of learning, wherever it takes place, and provide links between individual and organisational requirements: this should enable cost effective education and training programmes to be delivered.

The key to 'fitness for purpose' and 'fitness for practice' lies in the ability of Education Commissioners and Purchasers to reach agreement with the nurse education and training providers on the competence outcomes that a student should have acquired, and be able to use in practice, at the end of a nursing programme. (Storey *et al.* 1995) It is not inconceivable, therefore, to use National Vocational Qualifications (NVQs), national occupational standards and/or NVQ units as course outcomes, as these are part of a nationally accepted framework of qualifications and credit that focus on occupational competence. Although the achievement of vocational credit within nursing programmes can be used to meet the needs of purchasers in ensuring that staff are 'fit for purpose', it is essential that the requirements of statutory and professional bodies are also met within the programmes.

The issue of competence pervades all professional areas. Much work has been undertaken in the last few years to develop competencies or national occupational standards for professionals, these include accountants, engineers, psychologists, social workers, probation officers and health promotion advisors and professions allied to medicine.

NHS Executive funded projects have previously been commissioned to examine the relevance of national occupational standards to nursing. These include "Utilising National Occupational Standards as a complement to nursing curricula" (Storey *et al.* 1995) and "Occupational Standards - A Framework for Clinical Effectiveness?" (O'Hanlon and Andrews 1997) Both reports have concluded that occupational standards "have much to offer the nursing profession" (O'Hanlon and Andrews 1997), and suggest that national occupational standards "provide a common language that can be used to describe nursing and articulate clearly expected performance". They also provide a potential national curriculum template that would assist education providers in devising curricula, thus ensuring that nurses completing programmes are 'fit for purpose' (O'Hanlon and Andrews 1997).

This approach is becoming more common in the professional domain, as reported in the *Future Health Care Workforce*: "The professional bodies are increasingly aware of the need to deliver occupational competence. The Calman report on specialist medical training, for example states that the completion of specialist medical training should be based on assessment of competence...". (Conroy 1996)

Although there is a significant level of support for competence based approaches within the professional arena, there are critics of the processes involved. It is frequently the process of analysis and disaggregation of functions that has been criticised by a number of authors, including Le Var (1996) and Clark (1993). They suggest that this process is failing to meet the needs of nurses and nurse education. (Storey 1998)

Le Var (1996) critically examined the process of assessment associated with NVQs. She concluded that, "On the basis of research evidence of the effects of assessment on learning, assertions have been made regarding the likely effects of the NVQ approach to assessment on learning. These effects do not match the requirements of professional education and training aimed at producing a competent practitioner" (Le Var, 1996) This opinion reflects the views of other academics and professionals. Professor June Clark has stated that NVQs and Occupational Standards were potentially undermining professionals by reducing the qualifications required of them to a list of technical skills. Her major anxiety was that pre-registration education was slipping out of the profession's control. Another of Clark's worries was that professional education for nursing would gradually replaced by employer-led vocational training "a step back of more than 50 years". (Clark 1993) she also pointed out that preparation for nursing needs an intellectually stimulating, research-oriented, multi-disciplinary approach. "The socialisation process of the present vocational training system militates heavily against the creativity and intellectual curiosity...required for research and adaptability". (Clark 1993)

Storey (1998) refutes these views and suggests that these views demonstrate a lack of understanding of the processes involved in the development and implementation of national occupational standards and NVQs, and fail to acknowledge the changing needs of healthcare and education, and the policy direction being undertaken by the NHS Executive and the Department for Education and Employment. In Australia the Australian Nursing Council (ANC) has developed a framework of National Nursing Competency Standards (ANCI 1998) which are presented in a similar format to the national occupational standards utilised in the United Kingdom.

Competencies for Secure Environments

Robinson and Kettles (1998) suggest that the "forensic nurse is qualitatively different from the RMN owing to the nature of the client group and the environment". The scoping exercise confirmed that the client group and environment are significant factors to be considered. However the general view expressed by the majority of participants in the focus groups and interviews, was that the competencies, the knowledge skills and attitude, needed by nurses working in secure environments are the same as the RMN. The participants supported the view that their skills needed to be more finely honed, and they needed a greater understanding of the nature of the patients offending behaviour and the risk they present. Robinson and Kettles (1998) came to the conclusion that "the depth, quality, complexity and intensity of the therapeutic relationship over time and the level of security and control" are what distinguishes a forensic nurse from an RMN.

Some work has previously been undertaken to identify the competencies needed. In a study in Canada, the Registered Psychiatric Nurses Association of British Columbia (Niskala 1986 and 1987) identified the following core competencies:

- Maintain security
- Communicates effectively
- Maintain records and prepare reports
- Do counselling (sic)
- Perform the nursing process
- Plan and/or participate in programmes
- Conduct and participate in groups
- Perform and/or assist with diagnostic and treatment procedures
- Maintain professional role
- Carry out psychiatric nursing modalities
- Participate in research projects
- Instruct offenders, families and other staff
- Perform administrative functions.

These competencies seem to form the basis for of other frameworks, such as those developed by the Sainsbury Centre for Mental Health (1997), Watson and Kirby (1999), the University of Central Lancashire and Ashworth Hospital Authority (1997), the Standards in Forensic Social Work (CCETSW 1995) and the Core Competencies for Mental Health Workers commissioned by the NHS Executive North West Regional Office (1998).

The Sainsbury Centre identified a number of core competencies for mental health workers that have relevance for workers in secure settings. The 29 Core Skills are divided into 4 main areas:

- Management and Administration
- Assessment
- Treatment and Care Management
- Collaborative Working.

These generic core skills are being subject to further scrutiny and the Sainsbury Centre are currently in discussions with the National Training Organisations in Health Care and Personal and Social Care. The discussions are aimed at exploring the feasibility of developing National Occupational Standards for Mental Health Practice that would be applicable to all disciplines working in this field.

The State Hospital at Carstairs has developed competencies for maintaining a safe environment. The competencies are appropriate to all grades of nurses (Watson 1999). The competencies (Occupational Standards) were validated as S/NVQ units by SCOTVEC. The areas covered by the competencies include:

- Fire, searching, escorting, visitor control
- Risk assessment /management
- Assessment /management of dangerousness
- Prevention/management of aggression
- Observation, communication
- Management of hostage and other security breaches.

Occupational Standards have also been developed for delivering care and treatment including:

- Anger management
- Offence related work
- Reasoning and rehabilitation/moral reasoning and empathy
- Social skills training
- Psycho education
- Psychotherapies, counselling, PsychoSocial Interventions.

(Watson 1999)

The CCETSW competencies are also derived from occupational standards/competencies developed in other occupational areas that have then been contextualised for Forensic Social Work. A similar approach was taken by the University of Central Lancashire and Ashworth Hospital Authority who have developed a framework of occupational standards for staff

57

working with patients with a severe personality disorder. These standards reflect the needs of staff and patients in a secure environment. Although they were specifically developed for the multi-disciplinary team working in a Personality Disorder Unit they are readily generalisable and transferable to other nursing areas.

Development of Competency Framework

In the Prison Services nurses, need competencies associated with primary care as well as mental health care. This is consistent with the recommendation from *the Future Organisation of Prison Health Care* report that "there should be a focus on primary care within prisons and a move towards the establishment of primary care teams" (HM Prison Service and NHS Executive 1999). The report also suggests that "the role of nurses in prisons needs to be based on a more flexible and effective model of nursing competencies."

The competencies required for nurses working in secure environments are not clearly articulated by their employers. In the significant majority of cases the job descriptions for nursing posts described the main components of the job, including line of responsibility, but do not identify specific competencies. The job descriptions reviewed as part of the scoping exercise could be described as being Generic; they could apply to a wide range of posts in acute or secure settings. Generic job descriptions do not provide the post holder with a framework for their continuing development or to evaluate the effectiveness of an individual's practice. A small number of organisations are developing competence based job descriptions using competence frameworks from a number of sources.

In order to identify the competencies that were required to work in secure environments a number of approaches were taken. Individual interviews with managers, practitioners and educationalists were conducted, focus groups with practitioners from hospitals and the Prison Services were held and questionnaires from employing organisations and individual nurses were distributed and analysed.

From this data a number of key themes emerged. These were primarily in relation to relationships, boundaries, communication and counselling:

- safety and security,
- assessment and observation, including risk assessment and management
- management of violence and aggression, control and restraint, de-escalation techniques
- therapies and treatments, including Cognitive Behaviour Therapy and Psycho-Social Interventions
- knowledge of offending behaviour and appropriate legislation
- report writing
- "jail craft" (sic) (a term used to describe the prison context and culture)
- practical skills, including primary health care, first aid and "Practice Nursing"

These themes reinforce findings from other studies, including Niskala (1987) and the Sainsbury Centre (1997). The key themes were compared with the standards developed for staff working with personality disorder (University of Central Lancashire and Ashworth Hospital Authority 1997) and a framework of nursing competencies, or interventions, was developed for inclusion in the staff questionnaire. This framework reflected the need for competencies that meet both the mental and physical health needs of clients.

The nursing interventions (occupational standards) within the tool that was developed, were clustered into five key areas as follows:

1. Promote and implement principles which underpin effective, quality, practice
2. Assess, develop, implement, evaluate and improve programmes of care for individuals
3. Develop, implement, evaluate and improve environments and relationships which promote therapeutic goals and limit risks
4. Provide and improve resources and services which facilitate organisational functioning
5. Develop the knowledge, competence and practice of self and others.

(Storey and Dale 1998)

The finalised questionnaire was distributed to a total sample of nurses working in prison and to a randomised sample of nursing staff in the secure health sector (as previously described in Section 3.0 of this report). The 714 responses received from registered nursing staff working in prisons or health care have been analysed. (Appendix 5.5)

Analysis of Responses

Respondents' data were recoded to conflate responses for important and very important into one category "important"; and unimportant and very unimportant into one category "unimportant". Consequently, frequency analysis was computed using three categories, unimportant, undecided and important.

When asked whether the competencies were part of their role, respondents replied either that:
- the competency was or was not part of their role; or
- they were responsible for supervising others in relation to the competency.

A high proportion of respondents indicated that specific competencies were both part of their role and they were responsible for supervising others in carrying out this task. In the following section these responses have been combined and are represented in the bar charts as "part of role"

The items of data were analysed using the Statistical Package for the Social Sciences version 7.5 (SPSS). Firstly, competency statements were analysed to examine differences between the independent groups of the health sector and the criminal justice system (full details of frequency counts can be found in Appendix 5.5). The items of data were further cross tabulated to determine whether or not respondents recognised the competency as part of their role; and whether or not they regarded the competency as important. Statistical significance was examined by the Chi-square statistic incorporating the Yates's correction for continuity.

The competencies were clustered into groupings for clarity of reporting purposes.

The responses indicate that there is a clear endorsement that the competencies featuring in the staff questionnaire are, in the main, part of the role and are rated as important or very important by the majority of nurses in both sectors. From the 45 competencies there were 6 where less than 50% of nurses from the Prison Services said it was part of their role, whereas for hospital based nurses there was only one "Promote the needs of individuals in the community" which had less than a 50% response.

The six competencies with a low response rate in relation to being part of the role of nurses working in prisons were:

- Promote the needs of individuals in the community
- Negotiate, agree and support placements for individuals
- Develop, monitor and review discharge packages to manage individuals
- Enable individuals' partners, relatives and friends to adjust to and manage the individuals' loss
- Enable individuals, their partners, relatives and friends to explore and manage change
- Contribute to establishing and running mutual support networks

This response is not surprising as it may reflect the current role as understood by the majority of nurses working in prison.

The responses show a trend in relation to the level of importance attributed to the competencies. Hospital nurses tend to score the majority of competencies as being very important in contrast to nurses working in prison, who regularly rate the competencies as being important. One area where there is a variance from this pattern is in relation to meeting physical health needs, where nurses working in prison scored this cluster as being very important, again this is a reflection of role expectations and current education and training.

Another key finding on the analysis was the much higher reported level of both supervising and undertaking the role in the health sector. This was consistent throughout the competencies and was reported on average at over 3 times the level in health as in the criminal justice system. This finding may reflect the higher levels of skill/grade mix and numbers of nursing staff in the Health Service settings as compared to Prison Service settings. This situation has implications for the number of staff who would be expected to develop supervisory skills and to pursue the dual role of both supervising and directly providing clinical care.

Statistical Analysis

The individual competencies have been subject to a Chi-Square analysis and the statistical differences between responses from the prison services and health service are indicated as follows:

(NS)   Not significant
(S)   Significant (<0.05)
(HS)   Highly significant (<0.01)
(VHS)   Very highly significant (<0.001)

Two ratings are given against each competence, the first refers to "part of role" and the second to "level of importance"

(Complete tables of Chi Square results are included in appendix 5.5)
Clusters

Promoting:

Q 1	Promote people's equality, diversity and rights	S/S
Q 2	Promote effective communication and relationships	NS/NS
Q 3	Promote communication with individual where there are communication differences	HS/HS

Over 95% of nurses in both sectors agreed that they were part of the role and in excess of 90% rated them as important. There was a slightly increased score in each competency in favour of the health sector.

Assessing:

Q 4	Assess individuals to determine their overall needs and risk	NS/NS
Q 5	Provide specialist assessment services on individuals' needs so that others can take action	S/NS
Q 6	Assist in the assessment of, and the planning of programmes of care for individuals	S/NS

These three competencies concern the issue of assessment of patient needs for specialist services and assessment of risk. Both services recognised the need for a general involvement in determining overall needs and risks with 99.2% Health and 97.7% Prison service respectively (both sectors gave a slightly lower figure of level of importance - 93.9% and 92.9% respectively).

Fewer nurses viewed the provision of specialist assessment services, so that others could take action, as being part of their role, with 76.8% and 83.9% respectively stating that they did undertake this activity. These figures were also echoed in the results for level of importance, with 90.2% and 90.8% respectively.

In relation to the assistance in assessment of, and the planning of programmes of care for individuals, a high proportion of health sector nurses (99.6%) and nurses working in prison (97.2%) saw this as part of their role, with level of importance being 93.5 % and 91.7% respectively.

Enabling (1):

Q 7	Plan specific therapeutic interventions to enable individuals to recognise and address any socially unacceptable behaviour	VHS/VHS
Q11	Enable individuals to develop and maintain skills of independent living	VHS/HS
Q12	Enable individuals to develop to develop meaningful relationships with others	VHS/HS
Q13	Enable individuals who are at risk to themselves and others to identify behavioural boundaries and develop control	VHS/NS

These interventions relate to enabling individuals to address behaviours, develop skills of daily living and developing relationships. The health sector scored more highly in both, identifying the competencies as part of their role and in relation to the level of importance in relation to planning therapeutic interventions. This probably reflects the fact that these competencies have a stronger mental health bias which is not incorporated into the preparation of all nurses working in prison, particularly those on the General Part of the Register

Implementing:

Q8	Contribute to the joint implementation and monitoring of programmes of care for individuals	VHS/NS
Q 9	Implement specific therapeutic interventions to enable individuals to manage their behaviour	VHS/HS
Q 10	Assist in the implementation and monitoring of specific therapeutic interventions	VHS/HS
Q 14	Contribute to the evaluation and improvement of programmes of care for individuals	VHS/NS

Both sectors rated these competencies at over 85% important/very important. However, 26% and 17.9% of nurses working in prisons indicated that two of the competencies "Implement specific therapeutic interventions to enable individuals to manage their behaviour", and "Assist in the implementation and monitoring of specific therapeutic interventions" were not part of their role

Health & Evaluation of Primary Health Care Needs:

Q 15	Assess individuals' needs for primary health care services	HS/NS
Q 16	Develop, monitor and review programmes of primary health care for individuals	HS/S
Q 17	Contribute to raising awareness of health issues	NS/NS
Q 18	Enable individuals to address issues which affect their health and well-being	NS/NS

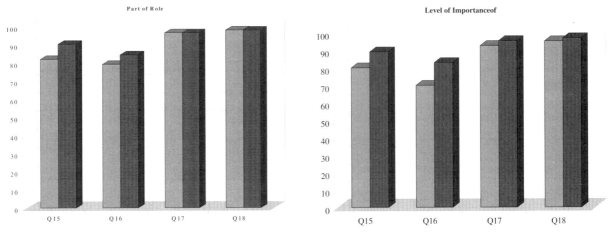

The competencies in relation to Health and Evaluation of Primary Health Care Needs appear to be of greater importance to nurses working in the Prison Services. The most notable differences were in relation to the assessment of individuals' needs for primary health care services (Health 82.1%; Prison Services 90.4%), and the development, monitoring and review of programmes of primary health care for individuals (Health 74.5%; Prison Services 84.5%).

This scoring reflects the greater input into meeting the physical health care needs of prisoners that nurses working in prison have as opposed to hospital nurses whose emphasis leans towards meeting mental health needs.

Discharge:

Q 19	Raise awareness of the needs of individuals discharged from your services	**NS/NS**
Q 20	Promote the needs of individuals in the community	**NS/NS**
Q 21	Negotiate, agree and support placements for individuals	**VHS/S**
Q 22	Develop, monitor and review discharge packages to manage individuals	**VHS/NS**

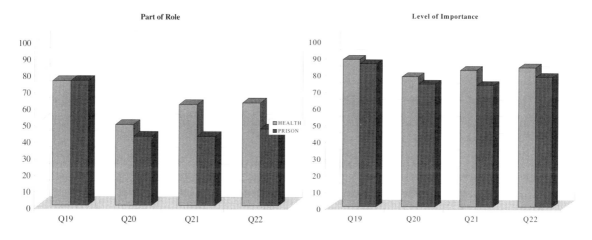

The lowest scoring of all competencies from both sectors was found in relation to discharge planning,

Of particular note was the lack of recognition for any on-going care, post discharge, for both health and particularly the Prison Services. In relation to the promotion of needs of individuals in the community, and the negotiation, agreement and support of placements for individuals the scorings were Health 48.2%, Prison 41.7%; and Health 61%, Prison 41.7%; respectively.

Although many nurses do not include these competencies as part of their current role a high percentage of staff, 73.4% hospital and 77.8% Nurses working in prison, felt that these issues were important and may reflect some of the organisational constraints and frustrations in role. It is worth noting that the *Future Organisation of Prison Health Care* report (HM Prison Service and NHS Executive 1999) suggests that action should be taken so that " at the end of a prison sentence adequate assessment and plans for discharge should be carried out to ensure continuity of healthcare".

Relationships

Q 23	Contribute to the provision of effective physical, social and emotional environments for group care	**VHS/VHS**
Q 24	Build and sustain relationships with individuals to reinforce their therapeutic goals	**VHS/VHS**
Q 26	Support individuals with difficult or potentially difficult relationships	**HS/HS**
Q 31	Contribute to establishing and running mutual support networks	**S/NS**
Q 32	Support individuals when they are distressed	**NS/NS**

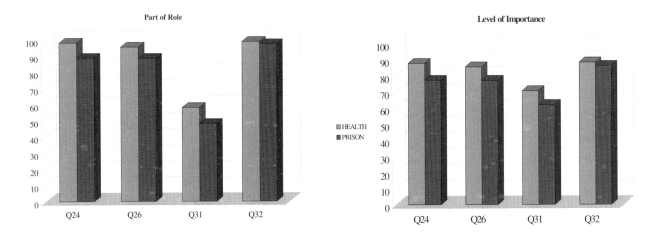

Both sectors identified relationships as a key part of their role and scored highly in relation to its level of importance.

One competency, however, in relation to contributing to the establishment and running of mutual support networks, scored poorly for both sectors, and was less enthusiastically supported in relation to level of importance.

Given the types of problems patients present with in both sectors (drug abuse, offences, self-injury), it is surprising that more importance is not given to the role of developing support networks. 77% of hospital nurses and 72.4% of Nurses working in prison rated this activity as important/very important. Although, this could reflect the view that patients in these settings are discouraged from developing networks because of the potential for concerted action against the institution. In many jurisdictions around the world great effort is put into preventing the development of sustained inmate relationships.

Safety:

Q 25	Physically intervene in situations where there is a breakdown in environments and relationships to limit risks to those involved	**VHS/VHS**
Q 33	Create and maintain boundaries between the community and individuals detained in secure conditions	**VHS/NS**
Q 34	Protect patients from themselves and each other	**VHS/NS**
Q 35	Contribute to the protection of individuals from abuse	**HS/NS**
Q 36	Escort patients within and beyond secure settings	**VHS/VHS**

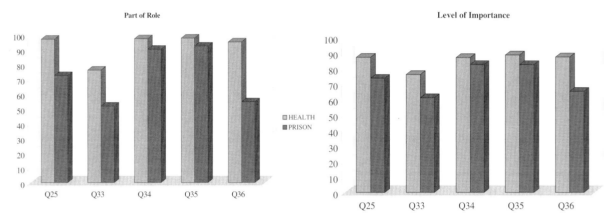

The data collected from the focus groups and focused interviews together with the staff questionnaire data indicates that the balance between therapy and security is the most consistently reported dilemma for nurses in all forms of secure care. However differences in role and responsibility are evident from the responses to the questionnaires.

The health sector respondents saw the physical intervention in situations where there is a breakdown in environment and relationships to limit risks to those involved, as a much more significant part of their role than the nurses working in prison (97.1% and 72.5% respectively). This finding is also reflected to a lesser extent in the level of importance that both sectors attributed to this competency.

A significant differential was also found between health and prison respondents in relation to the creation and maintenance of boundaries between the community and the individuals detained in secure conditions. The health sector scored this at 76.2% compared to 51.7% in the prison setting. (Similar percentages of 81.9 % and 75.8% respectively were found for the level of importance attributed to this). This result may reflect not only the category and security level of patients and inmates, but also the higher emphasis and use of physical security measures in the prison setting as opposed to the health sector. This reliance on physical security was seen in the High Security service before the more liberal policies of the early 1990's. (Fallon 1999) The realisation of the need to develop and enhance de-escalation skills has become more evident in the health sector, particularly in relation to people with a personality disorder.

It was stated on a number of occasions that difficult patients were easier to manage in a prison setting with clearer rules in relation to transgressions and a greater array of sanctions available to control behaviour. In these circumstances the need for psychological skills in relation to boundaries may be seen as less necessary.

The protection of individuals from each other and from abuse was seen as both a recognised part of role in a high percentage of cases (Health 97.4%, Prison 90.3%) and of high importance (Health 92.5%, Prison 90.6%) in both sectors.

The issue of escorting patients within and beyond secure settings was a much higher recognised role within the health service compared to the prison setting (95.2% and 54.6% respectively). This finding was also reflected in the level of importance attributed to this from both sectors (88.2% and 61.6% respectively).

This finding may reflect the type of escorts undertaken in. In the health sector this would be regarded as a key rehabilitation task that most nurses, particularly Primary nurses would undertake. In the Prison Services, health staff would not be participating as much in rehabilitative work but would be involved in out patient accident and emergency opportunities. Unsurprisingly therefore they see this as a much less important part of their role.

Enabling (2):

Q27.	Enable individuals to maintain contacts in isolating situations	**VHS/VHS**
Q28.	Enable individuals to adjust to and manage their loss	**S/NS**
Q29	Enable individuals' partners, relatives and friends to adjust to and manage the individual's loss	**VHS/VHS**
Q30	Enable individuals, their partners, relatives and friends to explore and manage change	**VHS/VHS**

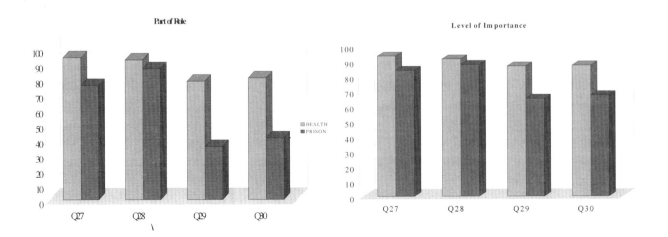

Again a high proportion of nurses in both sectors accept these competencies as part of their role. In the health sector 94.1% and 75.7% of Nurses working in prison see enabling individuals to maintain contact as being part of the role and being important. This was also reflected in the level of importance.

Health service nurses (92.5%) and nurses working in prison (86.7%) acknowledged that enabling individuals to adjust to loss is part of their role, and was important.

The scorings in relation to enabling individuals' partners, relatives and friends to adjust to and manage the individual's loss and change both reflect a lower level of involvement for the nurses working in prison in relation to families. Over 65% did not see this as part of their role. The health sector nurses however reported a 78.4% and 80.5% response to part of role and attributed a high level of importance to it (86.6% and 87.1% respectively). The prison nursing scoring,65.0 and 67.1 for level of importance raises questions of whether there should be greater opportunities for nurses working in prison to liase with families and friends of patients in their care, and contribute to a Care Planning Approach that includes throughcare.

In support of this view, Sir David Ramsbottom of HM Inspectorate of Prisons has stated that "all prisoners should strengthen links with their families and prepare for release". (HM Inspectorate of Prisons 1999)

Managing:

Q37.	Manage one's caseload against the prioritised needs of individuals	NS/NS
Q41.	Promote, monitor and maintain health, safety and security in the workplace	S/NS
Q42	Receive, transmit, store and retrieve information	NS/NS

In relation to these three competencies, both sectors responded with similar scoring for both part of role and level of importance. The lowest scoring of the three for both role and level of importance was in relation to the management of one's caseload against the prioritised needs of individuals (Health 86.2%, Prison 80.6%; and Health 87.1%, Prison 83.6%; respectively).

The competencies in relation to the promotion, monitoring and maintenance of health, safety and security in the workplace as well as the receiving, transmitting, storing and retrieval of information, scored highly for both part of role and level of importance in both sectors.

Supporting:

Q38	Support and lead teams to enable work objectives to be met	VHS/VHS
Q39	Support staff in maintaining their identity and safe personal boundaries	VHS/VHS
Q40	Counsel and support staff in times of stress	VHS/VHS

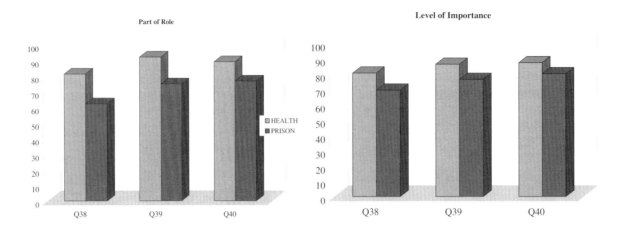

Supporting and leading teams was recognised as a role component for 81.5% of the health sector and a more modest 62.4% in the prison sector. These figures were slightly improved when reflected in the level of importance of this issue (90.5% and 86.7% respectively). This scoring may reflect the level of team development in both the health sector and particularly in the prison sector. Feedback from other sources would suggest that teamwork varies enormously between sectors, and also within services. It was not unusual to find examples of both good and bad practice at the same hospital with different teams operating.

The support of staff in maintaining their identity and safe personal boundaries was regarded as a more recognised role component in the health sector (92.3%) compared to the Prison Services (75.1%). These figures were also reflected in the level of importance attributed to this competency (Health 94.5 and Prison 92.8%). This finding reinforces the earlier observation in relation to higher level of and dependence on physical security in the prison sector as opposed to the health sector. It would be valuable to test this competency in a more open prison setting such as HM Prison at Grendon Underwood. This prison is unique in that it has five wings which are run as Therapeutic Communities each housing 40 prisoners who have been diagnosed as having a personality disorder The Prison has a twin role, as a prison and as a therapeutic facility which would equate more closely with a health sector secure environment.

The counselling of staff in times of stress was seen as a more recognised component in the health sector (89.3%) than in the prison sector (76.9%). These figures were also similar in the level of importance each sector placed on this competency (Health 94.1% and Prison 92.2%). This result may reflect the higher level of psychiatric trained staff in the health sector and the more generally accepted need to support staff psychologically in this sector.

Developing:

Q43	Contribute to the development of knowledge and practice	**HS/NS**
Q44.	Develop oneself within the role	**NS/NS**
Q45	Contribute to the development of others	**S/NS**

The findings across the development competencies were consistent across both sectors. Both sectors recognised that contributing to the development of knowledge and practice was a part of their role (Health 99.3% and Prison 95.5%) and was an important aspect of their role (94.9% and 93.3% respectively). Similar results were found in relation to the development of oneself within the role (Health 99.3% and Prison 98.1%) and its level of importance (94.3% and 94.5% respectively).

The contribution to the development of others was 96% for health staff and 90.8% for prison staff. These figures were also reflected in relation to the level of importance both sectors gave to this item (94.5% and 92.8% respectively).

In both sectors practitioners identified that it was an important part of their role to be involved in the development of themselves and others.

A comparison of responses from high and medium secure settings

Regional Secure Units were established to offer a new and alternative form of secure service from the Special/High Secure hospitals. These Regional Secure Units were later expanded and now include the independent sector and have been renamed medium secure units. Special hospitals have now been renamed as the High Secure hospitals. These new regional/medium secure services were seen to be less institutionalised, and without the constraining historical legacies of the special hospitals. Moreover, it was anticipated that different systems and potentially different roles may emerge for nursing staff. Therefore, it was decided here to also compare competency data for statistical significance between these independent groups; i.e., high and medium secure unit data within the health sector independent group.

One significant difference emerged between these two independent groups (high and medium secure units) for the level of importance placed on competencies by respondents. Even then, "develop oneself within the role", showed only a marginal difference between high and medium secure units (respectively 98.6% as opposed to 92.2 %); although both sectors clearly scored the competency at a high level of importance ($\chi^2 = 4.218$, df = 1, p<0.05). A full table of the Chi-square results can be found in Appendix 5.5

Seven significant differences emerged between high and medium secure unit respondents regarding whether the competencies were performed as part of their current role. These are as follows:

- a highly significant difference for "raise awareness of the needs of individuals discharged from your services" ($\chi^2 = 7.431$, df=1, p<0.01).
- a highly significant difference for "promote the needs of individuals in the community" ($\chi^2 = 10.228$, df=1, p<0.01).
- a highly significant difference for "negotiate, agree and support placements for individuals" ($\chi^2 = 8.027$, df=1, p<0.01).
- a very highly significant difference for "develop, monitor and review discharge packages to manage individuals" ($\chi^2 = 14.328$, df=1, p<0.001).
- a highly significant difference for "enable individuals' partners, relatives and friends to adjust to and manage the individual's loss" ($\chi^2 = 9.844$, df=1, p<0.01).

- a highly significant difference for "enable individuals, their partners, relatives and friends to explore and manage change" ($\chi^2 = 9.141$, df=1, p<0.01).
- a very highly significant difference for "create and maintain boundaries between the community and individuals detained in secure conditions" ($\chi^2 = 13.579$, df=1, p<0.001).

In all seven of the competencies showing these significant differences it was in the medium secure services that the higher percentages were found i.e. more nurses in these services identified these competencies as part of their role. Furthermore, all involve the interface between the service and the wider community; and four of the competencies involve discharging people into the community. This is an understandable difference between these two groups as medium secure units have a more active role and involvement with discharge directly into the community, whereas, this remains a relatively rare occurrence in high secure settings. Nurses in high secure settings may be involved in rehabilitation activities including escorts into the community, although, this is usually as preparation for moving patients to lower levels of security rather than preparing patients for discharge into the community.

Two competencies concerning working with the partners, relatives and friends of patients were identified as highly significant. This could be explained by high secure services having a less well established interface for nursing staff with patients' families and friends. For example, many patient visits take place in central visiting areas away from the ward environment and nursing staff including primary nurses may have limited contact with visitors. There are poorly developed systems in high secure care for therapy to embrace the wider family unit than is true in medium secure settings, some of which may reflect there geographic remoteness from the population they serve and also the low level of involvement in discharge preparation already identified.

The competency "create and maintain boundaries between the community and individuals detained in secure conditions" was scored more highly by Medium Secure Unit staff and is very highly significant when compared to High Secure settings. This response is possibly explained by the fact that patients in MSU's are more likely to interact within the local community than patients in High Secure services. Some of the High Secure services have explicit protocols that preclude the use of local communities for rehabilitation purposes.

Findings

The introduction of competence based job descriptions would enable employers and employees to have a clear understanding of expectations from both sides. This development could also impact on training needs analysis, individual performance review and provide a basis for developing continuing education packages that meet the needs of the service and individual employees.

The development of a competence framework would enable the sectors to identify the competencies needed to meet the demands of the service and to use the framework when negotiating with education providers to develop education and training tailored to the needs of the service.

The competence framework lends itself to the development of modular, competence based programmes that can be delivered through a number of media. Classroom based programmes do not need to be the main method of delivery, open and distance learning packages are available or can be developed.

The benefits of this type of approach are that modular programmes can be undertaken over a period of time and can therefore be more cost effective for participants. They can be multi-disciplinary in nature covering aspects of roles common to a range of health care professionals; multi-sectoral providing for the needs of both health care and the Prison Services. They also allow progression that will enable participants to undertake appropriate modules and achieve accreditation for completed modules; have multiple entry and exit points, again meeting the needs of individuals and employers. This approach acknowledges previous experience and qualifications and is flexible, and can thus be modified to meet changing needs.

The findings of this study indicate a high level of support for the competencies tested as both part of current role and in their level of importance. With the level of support and identification these competencies have received, they now provide a valuable starting point for the services to look towards developing job descriptions, training interventions and staff development utilising these as a framework.

It would be additionally useful to examine existing curricula for education and training programs relating to working in secure environments. A number of programs already validated by the National Boards and Universities could benefit from the incorporation of outcome based standards.

Conclusions

A competency framework was developed which built on existing work. It was modified in light of the focus groups and focus interviews and tested through the practitioner questionnaire.

As a result the following issues were identified:

- Competency based approaches offer a good model for developing practice in all secure environments.

- The competencies tested in the scoping study have received support as a framework on which to base future work.

- The results of this exercise demonstrate that there are significant areas of commonality in competencies between the Prison Services and the Health Sector

- The findings provide a basis for each sector - prisons and secure mental health care -to define more clearly the role responsibilities and competency expectations of nurses and for preparing competency based job descriptions.

- The competencies could be utilised to facilitate the development of modular, multi-disciplinary and cross-sectoral qualifications between Prison Services and Health Sector

71

- Differences in role competencies between the two sectors were identified in discharge planning, physical health needs, escorting, therapeutic approaches (individual and group), teamwork and support, maintaining relationships and client family/care contacts, all of which would benefit from further exploration.

4.2   Are Nursing interventions in secure environments evidenced based?

Evidence based practice can be viewed as a method of problem solving which involves identifying the clinical problem, searching the literature, evaluating the research evidence and deciding on the intervention. (Rosenberg and Donald 1995)

The theory-practice gap in nursing has been referred to in the past as a problem for nurses, both for those in academia and those in clinical practice (Thomson 1998). The phrase "theory practice gap" itself is open to a number of interpretations. It can mean theory driving practice, in that theoretical propositions are employed in practice; the second interpretation is that theories are formulated according to what happens in practice or thirdly all practice embodies theories and it is impossible for them not to do so. The use of evidence based practice in nursing is an attempt to take research findings and using them to guide practice, it is not just about applying theories

In relation to mental health issues, McKenna (1995) states that "people with mental health disorders deserve a service which has been demonstrated through research to be the best that can be given". He also notes that frequently the results produced by research are then not used in practice. Cutcliffe (1998) suggests that "The drive towards evidence based practice is one of the current issues facing mental health nurses ... Many mental health practitioners are engaged in generating this evidence..."

The quality of nursing research has improved. Davis (1981, 1986 and 1990) cited in McKenna (1995), has noted the progression of research in mental health nursing. McKenna (1995) also extracted four notable points from the examination: i) studies have increased in number, ii) they demonstrate a greater theoretical orientation, iii) they show a greater sophistication in their use of research methods, and iv) they have become more clinically focused. McKenna then notes however the minimal effect this has had on practising mental health nurses.

If nursing is to be evidence based then it will be necessary for a mechanism to be in place that allows and encourages them to pursue this goal. Evidence based practice (EBP), derived from general medicine, is one approach being taken to develop nursing practice. Whilst the National Institute for Clinical Excellence (NICE), Clinical Standards Advisory Group (CSAG) and Committee for Health Improvement in England, and the Clinical Standards Board and the Clinical Resource and Audit Group, in Scotland, are welcome recent developments, additional energy will be required at a local and operational level to ensure an uptake and consequential change in practice.

Flemming (1998) suggests evidence based nursing is a five stage process:

i)   information needs from practice are converted into focused structured questions
ii)   the focused questions are used as a basis for literature searching in order to identify relevant external evidence from research
iii)   the research evidence is critically appraised for validity and generalisability
iv)   the best available evidence is used alongside clinical expertise and the patient's perspective to plan care
v)   performance is evaluated through a process of self reflection, audit or peer assessment.

Evidence based nursing is a process that should make it easier to incorporate current best evidence into clinical decision making.

Sackett *et al.* (1996) are aware that the clinician is responsible for the decision making and that practice cannot be based purely on research. Nursing is not an exact science and frequently involves complex relationships between nurse and client. It would be difficult to dissect accurately this relationship into scientifically measurable items for research. Nursing can be unrealistically and inappropriately driven by evidence without an experienced clinician to guide it. However, to remain up to date and to use good new ideas, and to avoid becoming fixed in traditional routines, the best evidence from research is necessary. Cutcliffe (1998) suggests that "qualitative research could mean significant benefits for mental health nurses. If one accepts the argument that many of the interventions of mental health nurses are unmeasurable and invisible, then these nurses may well have difficulty articulating not only what they do, but also how worthwhile and valuable their interventions are... Qualitative studies can provide the methods by which the uniqueness of mental health nursing can be explored and understood more fully and provide data and theory to substantiate this argument". (Cutcliffe 1998)

Walsh (1998) attempts to describe what is meant by evidence and how an interpretation of evidence has also to take account of what is meant by clinical decision. If Evidence Based Nursing (EBN) is to be implemented successfully then for each patient the diagnosis must be accurate, the clinical plan effective and appropriate, and that the evaluation of the action objective (Walsh 1998). Clinical evidence therefore consists of contestable facts, experience and information offered to support the distinct claims that a clinical course of action is intelligible, truly effective, morally acceptable and sincerely intended (Walsh 1998).

Although randomised controlled trials (RCT) are seen as the 'Gold Standard' for systematic reviews, there is acceptance that it should not be the only source of evidence. It is recognised that in mental health RCTs are particularly difficult to apply and much of the research evidence in this field is qualitative (Mitchell 1998). EBN is concerned with finding the best evidence, if RCTs are not available then the next best external evidence should be sought. Once obtained, the evidence from research should be combined with individual clinical expertise before being applied.

The RCT frequently offers only statistical generalisability that is not appropriate to many situations faced by a mental health nurse attempting to gain knowledge about the individual and not the group (Rolfe 1998). If nursing care is based on research findings that offer the best overall care for a particular client group there is a danger in not meeting the needs of those that do not fit into the group exactly.

Mental health nursing appears to produce fewer examples of research than adult nursing that has been described as contributing to EBN. Much of the mental health evidence is concerned with diagnosis and prognosis. Typical of this is a review on suicide as an outcome for mental disorders (Sakinofsky 1997), another that looked at the prognosis for people with a diagnosis of borderline personality disorder who receive treatment in a therapeutic community (Cornah *et al.* 1997).

Incorporating research into practice involves a decision making process and there is an assumption that the process of making a decision is obvious (Walsh 1998). Walsh defines clinical decisions as clinical actions aimed at mastering clinical situations. Benner (1984) suggests that more experienced nurses incorporate their knowledge of research evidence into practice by using their own expertise and sometimes allow their own experience to override the scientific evidence. Inexperienced nurses however tend to uncritically rely more strictly on research evidence.

For EBP to become an integral part of nursing there is a need not just for educationalists, clinicians and researchers to adopt new approaches, but also for organisations. The emphasis on Clinical Governance means that organisations must make a commitment to provide time and staff, not only to the development of EBP, but also for the associated activities of quality assurance, clinical audit, staff development and job descriptions containing duties relating to research. (Royle and Blythe 1998)

Geddes *et al.* (1997) suggests that the recent increase in the amount of published literature in mental health nursing has rarely been reflected by changes in practice. There are several factors that are thought to influence the utilisation of research-based knowledge by nurses. However, MacGuire (1990) highlights the irony of this situation, in that, many of the reasons given as to why nurses fail to use research are not in themselves supported by research. As Bircumshaw (1990) comments in her review of the literature: "To summarise, most of the evidence to date has suggested that nurses do not utilise research in clinical practice. Most of this evidence has been anecdotal, personal experiences or opinions". This view was borne out during focus groups, focused interviews and the audits

Indeed, many of the articles that were found during the literature search were opinion based. This is not to say these articles and reviews do not make a valuable contribution to the general debate on the problem, but they offer few evidence-based solutions to the practitioner.

The research papers and articles that have examined research utilisation by nurses (by using the research process) conclude that there are four main factors that influence this process in clinical practice. These can be described as access, attitude, institutional support and occupational culture (see for example, Hunt 1987, Walczak *et al.* (1994), Champion and Leach 1989) added the concept of research utilisation. "This (research utilisation) means that research findings are used to define new practices and research methods are used to assist in implementing new practices with accuracy and in evaluating their impact on patients and staff". (Crane 1985)

Other authors have described two distinct strands of research utilisation. The "enlightenment" (Bulmer 1987) or "conceptual" model (Dunn 1983) is the more diffuse utilisation of research findings, which can indirectly inform policy or generally change the way in which an individual conceptualises a situation. In contrast, the "instrumental" (Dunn 1983) or "engineering" model (Bulmer 1987) is the direct application of research findings by a problem solving approaches "A problem exists, information or understanding is lacking either to generate a solution to a problem or to select among alternative solutions. Research provides the missing knowledge and a solution is reached.... policy makers and researchers agree upon what the desired end-state should be. The role of research is to help in the identification and selection of appropriate means to reach that goal". (Bulmer 1987)

The continuum starts with "research awareness - where a critical enquiring approach to practice is taken and questions raised about the rationale behind day-to-day practices" and moves to "Research activity - where a clear research question has been identified and becomes the subject of formal enquiry". (Vaughan and Edwards 1995)

Findings

The response from organisations indicated that there was a high proportion, 85% of health and 74% of prisons, used research findings in developing nursing practice. However, when asked to provide examples of evidence based practice, very few were able to produce examples that would meet the criteria discussed previously.

The utilisation of evidence within nursing in secure environments is affected by a number of factors:

- Access to information to inform practice
- Attitude
- Institutional support
- Occupational culture
- Diagnosis

Access to information to inform practice

Access not only refers to the availability of research findings from a library, newsletter and Journal Club, etc., but also to the ease with which findings can be translated into operational guidelines for practice. It also refers to the nurse's ability to understand and critique research-based information. Time, or to be more precise, lack of time for seeking out research findings and implementing them in practice could also be included here.

While conducting the Scoping Exercise the following data were collected, from the 714 nurses which identifies the extent to which nurses access to libraries on site and to up to date literature, and whether journals were delivered to the ward, data on the number of journals read was also captured.

	Access to library on site	Journal delivered to ward
Health	82%	46.3%
Prison	43%	75.6%

Table 4.2.1 Access to library and journals

As can be seen from the table above a higher percentage of hospital based nurses have direct access to a library on site, whereas a higher percentage of nurses working in prison have a professional journal delivered to their workplace.

	None	1-5	5 or more
Health	0.4%	25.4%	73%
Prison	3%	32.2%	64.1%

Table 4.2.2 Number of items of professional literature read in last 12 months

The majority of nurses in the survey had read 5 or more items of literature relating to their work whilst only 0.4% (*n=1*) of hospital nurses and 3% (*n=13*) nurses working in prison had not read any professional literature in the last twelve months

In a large survey undertaken by Pettengill *et al.* (1994) to ascertain factors encouraging and discouraging the use of nursing research findings, the authors concluded that lack of time was ranked as the main discouraging factor by nurse educationalists and service nurses. This result was found to be consistent with the findings of Funk *et al.* (1991) and Miller and Messenger (1978).

Barnard (1980) highlighted this issue, by stating that in many instances a time lag exists between the conduct of research and the dissemination of findings.

Another problem relating to access is the amount and quality of research-based information. For some areas, such as pressure area care, there is clearly an information overload Kim (1993), yet for others, there is a paucity of research-based literature and this seems particularly pertinent given the low level of forensic nursing research.

Very few of the educational providers in this survey reported any current research programmes underway into nursing in secure environments. Four respondents in total reported positively on this item representing 15% of all respondents

The topics covered by the research programmes reflected some of the current interest in the field of personality disorder (with two respondents reporting research in this area) and the continuing challenging area of working with women detained in secure settings. The final area of research covered multi-disciplinary working (see Table 4.3.3.below).

Title of Research Programme	N
Treatability of Personality Disorder	2
Education and Training needs of Staff Working with Women Patients	1
Multidisciplinary Working	1

Table 4.23 Topics covered by research programmes

This is undoubtedly a disappointing return given that all respondents were from the Higher Education sector. This may provide a fruitful area of closer co-operation between service and educational providers for mutually supportive research and education programmes, which could feed both into the practical and theoretical setting. It is difficult to see how a body of knowledge for nursing within these settings can emerge without a clear strategic approach in relation to the critical area of research.

Attitude

Attitude refers to the thoughts, feelings and actions nurses may have towards standards utilisation and research in general. Mahood (1995) described mental health nurses' 'phobic reaction' to research. This appears to be related to the belief that to 'do' research the nurse must be good at 'maths'; research being equated with something which incorporates a lot of 'confusing' statistics.

It has been shown in several studies that some nurses do not undertake regular professional reading, to update themselves on current practices based on research or development (Myco 1980, Webb and Mackenzie 1993). Professional reading and regular updating has traditionally been alien to nursing culture. Moreover, it is only since 1998, with changes in legislation that regular updating has become a statutory requirement for nurses. (UKCC 1998)

Several researchers have discussed the importance of a positive attitude towards research, and its relationship with research utilisation, both here and in North America. In a British study conducted by Lacey (1994), a positive correlation was found between attitude and research utilisation and across the Atlantic, similar results were found by Champion and Leach (1989). Attitude is only part of the problem. "The main findings suggest that although the vast majority of nurses in the study have a very positive attitude towards research, very few actually make significant use of research findings to enhance their clinical practice". (Veeramah 1995)

Accounting for these findings, Veeramah (1995) concluded that "Some of the variables that seem to contribute to this state of affairs are: lack of the necessary research appreciation skills to critically evaluate research findings and apply them in practice; not enough relevant research studies available in the clinical areas; and inadequate support from managers".

Institutional Support

The importance of institutional support for nurses attempting to utilise research-based knowledge is frequently commented on. In those projects where successful outcomes have occurred, institutional support was a key feature.

Horsley *et al.* (1983), cites a high profile committee of senior nurse managers who identified areas of practice with a sound research base and then co-ordinated the practice innovations at ward level.

Hunt (1987) argued, "If changes in practice are warranted it is not sufficient to inform staff and leave ward sisters or qualified practice, staff to be autonomously responsible for making changes. As has been demonstrated, changing inappropriate organisational contexts and resources and negotiating with a range of disciplines are generally beyond the capacity of one individual".

Institutional support also refers to the rewards and reinforcement nurses receive for utilising research-based knowledge in practice. Out of the 215 nurses surveyed in Miller and Messenger's (1978) study, just under half, 42% indicated insufficient institutional rewards for using research.

Such rewards and reinforcement have been described as "time off for attending nursing conferences, availability of libraries with current journals, and time off for reading made available during the working day. In addition, nursing leaders who support the concept of research as well as staff nurses who support research within a service setting were considered important". (Champion and Leach 1989).

In a number of organisations the appointment of Clinical Nurse Consultants, Clinical Nurse Specialists and Research Nurses as well as joint appointments with Universities are noteworthy ways of formally establishing and recognising the role of clinical staff in relation to both the conduct and utilisation of research.

The conduct of clinical research depends upon institutional support, including the provision of appropriate staff development opportunities, material resources and encouragement. Unless these are forthcoming, clinical research in the field can not be expected to develop. Among the ways in which institutions inhibit research include the creation of bureaucratic barriers preventing access to sources of data, for example refusing to allow staff to conduct research during working hours, and denying access to case records, the creation of obstructive and over-protective research approval processes, the failure to routinely gather important data, and the failure to ensure that nurses and others keep accurate records. These are real disincentives for anyone wishing to carry out research in secure settings, and would tend to undermine the value of any that has begun.

Occupational Culture

One of the salient features of nursing in secure environments is that most of its members work in the closed society of the ward, and this in itself creates a unique occupational culture in each group in each and every ward. Research based practice obviously represents a great threat to occupational cultures. Not only does it represent something new, it also has as its guise the desire to eradicate 'old routines and rituals' and replace them with practices that are scientifically legitimated. There is little doubt that many advocates of research utilisation amongst nurses see occupational culture as one of the major barriers to effective change.

According to Walsh and Ford (1989) - nursing has traditionally been subservient to medicine, has lacked a unique body of knowledge of its own, and has by necessity relied heavily on medical knowledge, in the form of doctors' instructions.

Studies on organisational climate within nursing have demonstrated the powerful aspects of ward culture. Although not directly related to research utilisation, they have demonstrated how ward culture can facilitate or hinder the learning process for student nurses. 'Climate' refers to the social pressure exerted on an individual to conform and behave as expected by others in specific social environments. Several researchers have demonstrated in their studies the powerful effects on both patients and staff of the ward climate or culture (Melia 1987, Moos and Hout 1968).

The study by Melia (1987), in a high secure hospital, found that students have to 'fit in' and 'learn the ropes' on each ward setting they encounter. As a result, the more professional aspects of their work are abandoned in favour of the more physical and manual approaches to nursing, valued by the ward climate. Although participants in the scoping exercise suggest that there have been significant changes since then, and a more positive attitude is experienced by students.

It is not surprising therefore that research utilisation, entailing as it does, visits to the library, reading, discussion groups etc., will not be seen as a priority by many hard pressed nurses.

Reading research papers and undertaking literature searches became to be seen by many of the unqualified staff as 'slacking off ' (Gadd *et al.* 1995).

The Foundation of Nursing Studies (1996) has recently launched a report which reinforces the importance of understanding local research cultures. In the report's summary and implications, the Foundation states, "Dissemination and implementation strategies must be grounded in an appreciation of the complexity and social nature of research utilisation".

There are many expectations being made on registered nurses today, regarding the utilisation of research-based knowledge, but it must be remembered that nursing has a relatively short history of both conducting and using research. If the statistical research by Florence Nightingale is ignored, the first known research published by a British nurse was that of Skellem in 1953, a leading figure in mental health nursing (Butterworth 1991). Moreover, the traditional apprentice style training of nurses has not enhanced nursing's academic credibility. It has only been with the introduction of Project 2000, that UK nurses have received an education rather than training. In addition, it is only over the past few years that this change in emphasis has largely been extended to post-registered nurses, through the English National Board's (ENB) Higher Award (ENB 1991). Whether or not this new breed of nurses can influence and change the culture within nursing, so that research-based practice becomes the norm remains to be seen.

Diagnosis

The nursing staff within the scoping exercise identified a major concern in relation to the issue of diagnosis, which was often in dispute and difficult to pinpoint, with many instances of mixed diagnosis. It was not unusual for these disagreements to be within the clinical teams caring for the patient. Irrespective of diagnosis the problems that these difficult patients generated for the system and the way that staff felt towards them had much in common. It is interesting to note the work of Maden *et al.* (1995), looking at the treatment and security needs of Special Hospital patients, they found that although the patients had a mixed diagnosis the management and care regimes were fundamentally similar, as indeed was this study's findings in relation to these difficult groups.

Given the problems of diagnosis, nursing staff also identified treatment issues as a cause for concern. There were often signs of friction and disagreement amongst clinical teams about the most appropriate approach to treatment. Some of this could be identified as a different philosophical approach, which was particularly true in the dichotomy between a behavioural approach and the psychodynamic, psychotherapeutic approach. This often left nurses in an invidious position of attempting to "square the circle" of appeasing competing demands.

The development of evidence based nursing practice in a secure environment

The dearth of evidence based practice is apparent in the literature reviewed. The literature search identified over 680 papers, articles, and book chapters and unpublished works relating to nursing in secure environments, the majority can be categorised as clinical anecdotes. Nursing research in this area appears to depend on "Opinion or Experience Based Practice". Many of the authors describe their experience of working with particular clients, explaining the nursing interventions used and give an opinion on the effectiveness of the intervention. In a number of the papers the opinions become shared opinions and it is difficult to say at what stage opinion based practice becomes evidence based.

Other phenomena that are emerging are "Incident Based Practice" and "Inquiry Based Practice". Incident Based Practice can be described as practice that emerges as the result of a serious incident encountered by an individual or organisation which result in changes in practice in order to prevent a reoccurrence of the incident. Inquiry Based Practice is similar in that an Inquiry has taken place as the result of an incident, the Inquiry Team have made recommendations and practice once more changes as the result.

Whilst both incident based and enquiry based practice are understandable, particularly in the highly sensitive and media pressured world of the secure environment, they bring with them attendant problems. These services, particularly the high secure hospitals and Prison Services, often have practices handed down as a consequence of some past incident or inquiry which the current staff have no direct knowledge of or reasons why they continue to exist. These changes can often be brought about in a reactive manner to pacify the general public, particularly in relation to security and control of risk. From an internal viewpoint professional and staff side organisations have also been a source of tremendous pressure for management to introduce change to protect members where they perceive a practice may be putting their members at an unacceptable risk.

The problem with some of these changes is they are not taken in an objective and considered way but often in the heat of the moment to meet agendas other than the evidence based care of individuals. Some of this can most graphically be illustrated by the variance between secure environments, particularly in the health sector, and what are considered to be banned items on security grounds. There are instances where items are permissible to be taken into one high secure environment or medium secure unit which are banned as a result of some incident in an identical unit dealing with similar patients with similar admission and discharge criteria. Once instigated, these changes often stick for many years as they become part of the folklore and day to day practice, and can remain unchallenged for many years. (Many anecdotal examples of this were related during the focus groups and focussed interviews.) A valuable exercise would be an objective evaluation of many of these incident and inquiry based practices with a view to a re-evaluation of their necessity and efficacy. These could in themselves lead to a development of standards for practice.

Perhaps the latest and most vivid demonstration of this came with the recent *Fallon Inquiry Report* (1999) held only six years after the previous public inquiry had examined the same hospital and at least in part, the same services. The *Fallon Inquiry Report* (Department of Health 1999) was clearly critical of the political response in light of the *Blom Cooper Report* (Department of Health 1992) and stated that the implementation of these findings had been ill-considered and had led to many of the problems which the Fallon Inquiry Report identified and reported on.

Practitioners, during the focus groups and interviews, reported that difficulties arise in these circumstances as they are clearly given blueprints and direction particularly from major reports such as this, only to find themselves criticised for carrying out the very acts that the original reports were based upon. From a nursing perspective, a sensible way forward in light of this is to establish an explicit agreement on what constitutes best practice and provide a robust defence of this agreement should it subsequently be called into question or threatened. It would also be helpful if official inquiries were not allowed to create a culture of blame and mistrust, and strategies could be mobilised which would reduce their harmful effects on staff morale.

Kaye and Franey (1998) state that "the hospitals and their staff work with little public support or understanding and, often with public criticism... The work is in the public eye and little distinction is made in that glare between taking measured risks, making mistakes or even unfounded rumours. All are likely to be pounced upon, headlined, condemned and abandoned before any response or evaluation can be properly made. An unforgiving public is impatient with explanation and justification. But the responsibility remains and with it the requirement to treat and to respond to individual needs."

A number of inquiry reports have identified the problems and difficulties in relation to policies and procedures, not least of which is their implementation in practice. It was very evident from our findings that there was inconsistency on the availability and evidence base for those policies and procedures that were currently available in practice. When they did exist, there was not a systematic way to ensure that staff read and understood these documents and in particular, they were poor mechanisms in ensuring that they were applied in practice.

Although the Scottish Prison Service developed and implemented a nursing philosophy in 1995, this is not the case across all of the Prison Services. One HM Prison Inspection report states that one of the prisons inspected had a written 'health care philosophy', which included the statement "care will be research based", this then went on to outline their aims, which are to be informed by relevant research and inquiry. Another reference to EBP was in a more negative light, "there were occasional references to women having abusive or deprived backgrounds, but very little evidence of this information being used to develop or inform any specific treatment approach". This is an ideal opportunity for the nurses involved to research this area and develop a relevant treatment strategy based on their findings." (HM Inspectorate of Prisons 1998)

Given the difficulties, described elsewhere, in relation to erosions of boundaries and the particularly challenging patient group being cared for in these environments, one way of ensuring consistency in practice is to ensure that the policies and procedures are adhered to. It would be a valuable resource to all secure services to have an agreed set of policies and procedures that they had confidence as being based in the best known evidence available. These should be subjected to systematic reviews and updates and form part of induction and continuing education to ensure there is appropriate knowledge and application in practice settings.

Conclusions

Over 680 items of literature, identified as relevant to the key themes, were analysed. Educationalists and Practitioners were asked through the questionnaires about access to evidence. Research by educationalists was reviewed.

The issues identified are:

- While there is significant literature on nursing in secure environments, this has not been subjected to a systematic evaluation that could result in the identification of an evidence base that could be applied to enhance practice.

- The published research evidence is generally derived from clinical anecdotes and concentrates on discussion rather than the presentation of empirical based data.

- There is clear evidence that nurses in secure environments, both in the Health and Prison sectors, have reasonable access to sources of evidence through libraries and professional journals.

- Even though nurses working in secure environments appear to believe that the standards they are expected to implement are evidence based, there is little evidence from the literature, survey questionnaires and audits to support this belief.

- Nursing today is based on the concept of reflective practice, but there is little evidence to show that nurses are reflecting on their current practice and implementing change in practice as a result

- Closed environments, in particular, are motivated, at least by part, by a reliance on 'routines, rituals and regimes'; evidence based practice appears to have difficulty penetrating this.

- Employers need to develop and maintain a culture in which nurses are enabled to subject their practices to scrutiny and make appropriate changes in light of current best practice.

- The evidence on which much nursing practice is shaped is 'Incident and Inquiry' based practice which derives from a risk management perspective. However, because of the limitations of this approach, developments in practice arising from it may become skewed towards containment rather than therapeutically orientated care.

- The political sensitivities relating to secure environments, and the media attention they attract, results in defensive reactions to incidents rather than a considered research based approach to the solution of problems.

4.3 Review Current Activity in the Development of Practice Standards in Secure Environments, Particularly With Reference To Specific Client Groups

Standards are authoritative statements by which the nursing profession, and thus forensic nursing, can describe the responsibilities for which its professionals are accountable. Consequently, standards reflect the values and priorities of the profession of and provide direction for nursing practice and a framework for the evaluation of its practice. Written in measurable terms, standards also illustrate the nursing profession's accountability to the public and the outcomes for which nurses are responsible. Standards of professional nursing practice may pertain to general or speciality practice.

The International Association of Forensic Nurses & American Nurses Association (1997) describes "Standards of Care" thus, "a competent level of forensic nursing practice as demonstrated by the nursing process, which involves assessment, analysis, outcome identification, implementation, and evaluation. The nursing process encompasses all significant actions taken by forensic nurses in providing services to all clients, and forms the foundation of decision-making. Additional nursing responsibilities for all clients, such as providing culturally and ethnically applicable services, maintaining a safe environment, and planning for continuity of care and services, are embodied within these standards. Therefore, "Standards of Care" delineates services that are provided to all clients of forensic nurses or practitioners."

In the United Kingdom, standards have been seen as an essential component of "Continuous Quality Improvement" which formed a cycle of Set Standards; Measure Standards (Audit), Review Standards, Action for improvement and repeat.

These standards are taken from:
- Professional and statutory codes of conduct and practice
- Service contracts with purchasers
- Health and Safety Standards
- NHS Patient's Charter
- Prison Health Care Standards

and, more locally:
- Clinical Audit programmes
- Complaints trends
- Patients representation
- Ward/departmental standard
- Incidents/Inquiries

"Standards of Professional Performance" describes a competent level of behaviour in the professional role, including activities related to quality of services, performance appraisal, education, ethics, collaboration, research, and resource utilisation. All nurses are expected to engage in professional role activities appropriate to their education, position, and practice setting.

One of the key characteristics of standards is their measurability. Criteria include key indicators of competent practice. For the most part, standards should remain stable over time, as they reflect the philosophical values of the profession. However, criteria should be revised to incorporate advancements in scientific knowledge, practice, research, and technology. Criteria must remain consistent with current nursing practice, which has a theoretical basis but is constantly evolving through the development of new knowledge and incorporation of relevant research findings into aspects of the nursing process.

The Standards of Clinical Nursing Practice focuses primarily on the process of providing nursing care and performing professional role activities. These standards apply to all nurses in all areas of clinical practice despite the tremendous variability in environments in which nurses' practice. However, it is important to recognise the link between working conditions and the nurse's ability to deliver services. It is the responsibility of employers or health care facilities to provide an appropriate environment for forensic nursing practice.

Well-articulated sets of standards could facilitate:
- Quality assurance systems
- Databases
- Regulatory systems
- Health care reimbursement and financing methodologies
- Development and evaluation of nursing service delivery systems and organisational structures
- Certification activities
- Job descriptions and performance appraisals
- Agency policies, procedures and protocols
- Educational offerings.
(The International Association of Forensic Nurses & American Nurses Association 1997)

In recent times standards have been developed and disseminated in the guise of clinical guidelines. Guidelines are "scientifically developed statements to assist practitioner and patient decisions about appropriate care for specific clinical conditions" (Field and Lohr 1992, cited in Cheater and Closs (1997)).

The NHS describes standards as, "the extent to which specific clinical interventions, when deployed in the field for a particular patient or population, do what they are intended to - i.e. maintain and improve health and secure the greatest possible health gain from the available resources" (NHS Executive 1996). The NHS Executive has supported the production of effective health care bulletins, epidemiological based needs assessments, clinical guidelines and systematic reviews of research evidence (NHS Executive 1996).

Guidelines are not intended to be prescriptive and compliance is intended to be guided by individual patient circumstances and preferences (Cheater and Closs 1997).

A systematic review of the effectiveness of clinical guidelines has shown that they can improve both the processes and outcomes of care in medicine (Grimshaw and Russell 1993a, Grimshaw et al.1995). There is also limited evidence that guidelines for nurses and professions allied to medicine impact positively on the processes and outcomes of patient care (Thomas et al. 1998).

The adoption of guidelines is not automatic and depends on a range of factors including how they are developed, disseminated and implemented (Grimshaw and Russell 1994, Freemantle *et al.* 1995, Grimshaw *et al.* 1995, Lewin *et al.* 1998). Findings from two surveys reported by Lewin *et al.* (1998) show that adherence to national guidelines (cardiac rehabilitation guidelines) is poor.

This problem of poor uptake of national and local standards has parallels in the poor uptake and implementation of research generally by nurses. The importance of understanding the local research culture, in relation to the implementation of research findings in nursing practice, has recently been highlighted in a national report (The Foundation of Nursing Studies 1996).

Not all clinical guidelines are based on sound research evidence. Some have been based on expert opinion or nationally accepted practice.

The formulation of clinical protocols involves the synthesis of research evidence into a format that can be used by practitioners. Each protocol focuses on a particular patient 'need' and the nursing actions related to it.

In Scotland, The Clinical Resource and Audit Group (1993) have clarified the utilisation of clinical protocols further, by making the distinction between the use of clinical guidelines and clinical protocols: "The distinction between protocols and clinical guidelines concerns the amount of operational information contained within each. Where clinical guidelines reflect a broad statement of good practice, with little operational detail, protocols are the result of their adaptation for use in the local context". (Clinical Resource and Audit Group 1993)

Although the use of clinical guidelines and protocols for transferring research-based knowledge into clinical practice are being advocated nationally, it is interesting to note that these methods have not been extensively evaluated or researched, to assess their effectiveness (Duff *et al.* 1996). The Department of Health, recognising this lack of research into research utilisation by nurses and other health professionals, has set twenty priority areas, to evaluate methods to promote the implementation of research findings in the NHS. Amongst these are (Department of Health, England: 1995):

1.   Why some clinicians but not others change their practice in response to research findings,
2.   The impact of clinical practice guidelines in disciplines other than medicine,
3.   The role of undergraduate (pre-qualification training) in promoting the uptake of research findings.

Findings

A detailed analysis was made of the results of 18 audits (9 Criminal Justice and 9 Health sector) which were conducted at all levels of the security spectrum of both services. The quantitative data from the focus groups, focused interviews and comments on the organisational questionnaires was also scrutinised for key themes, and issues, emerging in relation to the development of practice standards.

When reviewing services, evidence was sought to establish whether the ward team audited standards at least twice a year with any necessary changes implemented. This was found to be true in only 50% of cases, with a further 25% of services auditing standards on an annual basis.

Only 50% of the services visited displayed standards for patients' information and the general level of information routinely available to patient was disappointing.

Over 20% of services audited had no member of the ward team who had been instructed in standard setting and could therefore act as a resource to the team. Given the primacy of standard setting and development in quality management systems, this was a disappointing finding.

We asked the staff how satisfied they were with their involvement in the development of policies and procedures, and found that 60% of the nursing staff were dissatisfied. Policies and procedures have been highlighted repeatedly in inquiry reports, most noticeably in the recent report into the Personality Disorder Services at Ashworth Hospital (Fallon 1999), where both the knowledge of, and compliance with, policies and procedures was criticised. It cannot help the acceptance and uptake of policies and procedures if staff do not feel part of the process or feel able to influence this development.

Both sectors used the terms 'protocols', 'guidelines' and 'standards' interchangeably, and there was an apparent lack of clarity and understanding on the true meanings of the terms.

Specific standards were referred to by the nursing staff as either being in existence or in need of revising in relation to Epilepsy and Hepatitis A, B and C, specifically from the Prison Services. The Prison Services also laid great emphasis on detoxification protocols covering both drug and alcohol withdrawal; this was not a feature from the health sector.

Suicide and self harm featured frequently in both sectors and standards were stated to be in existence for most services, but it was not determined what level of contemporary practice these reflected. Both sectors made frequent reference to security and risk assessment management systems available as standards or in the process of development. Other examples cited included standards for:

- the provision of women's services
- chronic disease management, including asthma, diabetes and epilepsy
- management of communicable diseases, including HIV and AIDS, Hepatitis
- seclusion and special observations
- non-prescription medications

Two key areas which caused considerable concern for nurses in the Prison Services, were in relation to medication (particularly adherence to UKCC standards) and physical restraint of patients. Nursing staff felt vulnerable in potentially breaching the professional code of conduct in relation to both activities by the non-availability of clear standards that were capable of being consistently applied in practice.

The general issues that emerged from observation visits and meeting with a large cross section of staff was that there was evidence of pockets of good practice in standards development. The unfortunate aspect of this was that this work, often involving intense activity over a protracted period of time had not been shared beyond the confines of the service or the team developing it. Although a significant amount of work has been undertaken across the UK to develop standards there are still areas where the application and implementation of the standards could be improved.

Hunt (1981) suggests the five following reasons, as to why nurses do not use the standards or research findings in practice:

"They do not know about them;
They do not understand them;
They do not believe them;
They do not know how to apply them;
They are not allowed to use them."
(Hunt 1981)

Another factor that can be added to this list is "They do not own them". From the audits and focus groups it is apparent that nurses do not own many of the standards because they have not contributed to the development or implementation of the standards. It was also stated that organisations frequently "pay lip service" to involving "shop floor" staff in this process.

To a certain extent Hunt's findings were confirmed during the focus groups, focused interviews and audits. There are a number of instances cited where standards have been developed in one part of an organisation that were unknown to other wards or department on the same site. The same problem has been encountered within the Prison Services. Standards and protocols are being developed in some establishments to meet the needs of their client group but the outcomes of this work are not shared with colleagues in other prisons, or are not seen to be useful because the standards do not exactly fit the context of the organisation.

The Prison Service in Scotland has the benefit of being able to adopt a corporate approach to the development and implementation of standards for care. In England and Wales, standards are being developed and implemented in a number of Prisons and Hospitals but the identification and sharing of good practice amongst organisations and individual nurses in both sectors is haphazard. Good practice does not travel within some areas of these sectors. The development of networks to evaluate and disseminate good practice would have benefits to the delivery of quality healthcare.

Much of the work that did exist was not evidence based, what was often lacking was a reference to contemporary evidence on research literature and there was no systematic procedure in place for amending or updating standards in the majority of cases.

Linked to the confusion on terminology was the problem that few staff understood the purpose of standards or what could be achieved by their incorporation.

The production of central standards in the Prison Services, whilst in many instances laudable, has led to an over reliance on this system for the provision and setting of standards at a local level. An almost reflex response for nurses when quizzed about standards was to make reference to the manual. What failed to be recognised was that those standards themselves are not based on sound empirical evidence. This situation has also led nurses working in prison to an over-reliance on the centre for development and production of standards. It would make a more efficient use of skills and resources to see this as a partnership. There could be much mutual benefit in seeing the responsibility for the development and collation of standards to be a shared task.

Application of standards also varies from Prison to Prison according to priority accorded by the Governor. In England and Wales, *the Future Organisation of Prison Health Care* report has suggested that "Prisons should designate a clinician responsible for ensuring that clinical governance is in place and that regular reports are produced for the governor. As the head of the prison the governor is ultimately responsible for assuring the quality of services provided in the prison." (HM Prison Service and NHS Executive 1999) This statement has implications for nursing, as it will encourage a wider compliance to the prison health care standards.

The review of Prison Inspection reports for England and Wales, and Scotland provides further evidence that nurses have difficulty in applying the Health Care Standards. One report states that " the level of nursing staff available and on duty...were insufficient to provide an NHS equivalent standard of care..." (HM Inspectorate of Prisons 1998). Many references to this issue in other reports are as negative and there are already signs that professional standards are having to be 'bent' to prison directives. (HM Inspectorate of Prisons 1996) This can in turn cause difficulties for nurses aiming to implement practice standards because they may conflict with already existing prison policies.

The Inspectorate also report positive action, there was also evidence of the opposite side of the coin, where nursing care was not compromised - "the health care centre has a comprehensive set of policies, protocols and job descriptions". In another prison the Nurse Manager had identified the need "to promote professional competence" as an immediate priority. Whilst there are two variables (custody and care) at work in these environments, there can be little development and implementation of a comprehensive and relevant set of nursing practice standards.

Conclusions

The development of practice standards (clinical / practical and organisational protocols) was reviewed in both sectors. Examples were collected through the practitioner questionnaire. The focus groups provided considerable evidence in relation to the development and utilisation of practice standards.

- There could be early gain in targeting the sensitive and problematic areas for staff and working towards the joint production and implementation of standards, utilising external expertise and guidance where this was indicated.

- The production of standards is one task, then implementation and monitoring in practice is another. Routine and regular audit activity, training and education together with a clear expectation of staff reflected in the job descriptions would all be helpful adjuncts to their visibility in practice.

- Discussion with participants within the scoping exercise identified a need to determine national minimum criteria for locally developed policies and protocols. These might include policies and protocols in relation to security items, seclusion, leave of absence, and physical health monitoring.

- There is significant evidence of a wide range of practice standards having been developed in some aspects of secure care and the Prison Services.

- There is little co-ordination across and between services and there is poor dissemination and uptake of standards.

- There is little research evidence neither within these standards nor of quality control or validation of them.

- The auditing of standards across services is haphazard or minimal.

- There is significant evidence that practitioners feel that they bare excluded from the development of organisational standards

- The development of standards in many instances is a response to incidents or inquiries, rather than a pro-active strategy for meeting the needs of client groups.

- There is confusion among nurses, and their employers, about what "standards" are, particularly in relation to protocols and guidelines.

- There is significant evidence that practice standards are not made known to clients, and that clients have little input into the development of standards.

- The development and implementation of standards for health care needs to be supported within the Performance Indicators for an organisation and subjected to regular audit and up-date.

4.4 How effective is the preparation currently given to nurses working in secure environments?

The preparation of nurses to work in secure environments can be categorised into two main areas:
- pre-registration
- post-registration, including continuing professional development and induction into new roles.

Pre -registration

The pre-registration preparation of nurses has been subject to review from a number of authors. (Gilmore 1998, May *et al.* 1997, Eraut and Cole 1993) In the majority of cases these reviews relate to the generic preparation rather than for working in a secure environment. May *et al.* (1997), in their report into the branch and common foundation programmes of project 2000 courses found an over emphasis on theory within the programmes and that theory and practice were not linked. This coupled with the number of short placements available to students reduced their ability to develop the appropriate skills.

The English National Board guidance to education providers, 'Creating Lifelong Learners-Partnership for Care' highlights the need for students "to develop their skills and to gain the necessary confidence, they need to have experience of caring for people with a variety of mental illnesses across the age range. Examples include mentally disordered offenders, people who abuse substances...people with challenging behaviour" (ENB 1994).

The literature search also highlighted a number of key points. Although Reed's (1992) review examined issues in England, the results from the questionnaires and interviews shows that the issues are evident across the UK. In the report Reed made a number of recommendations including:

- that training courses for community psychiatric nurses include consideration of forensic nursing issues and opportunities for placement in forensic settings
- that the ENB considers the future need for Project 2000 training in forensic psychiatric nursing, including opportunities for suitable placements
- that prisons continue to forge closer links with local hospitals, colleges of nursing and others who can assist in the development of nurse education.

Reed also predicted that "it is likely that they (Project 2000 students) will have received rather less specialised training than their RMN and RNMH predecessors, while opportunities for practical experience of the range of problems found among psychiatric in-patients are increasingly limited due to the provision of services away from hospitals. It is reasonable to assume, therefore, that Project 2000 students would require some additional education in forensic psychiatric issues, although greater emphasis should now be given to such opportunities as part of post-registration training". (Reed 1992)

However, from an analysis of the research data, extracted from questionnaires completed by education providers, offering mental health and learning disabilities programmes, a significant variation has been found in this criteria being applied. Some education institutions provide an opportunity for students to undertake a 13 week elective in a secure environment, others include a shorter placement as an integral part of the mental health or learning disabilities branch, whilst some institutions only provide a single lecture on the issue of Mentally Disordered Offenders. In all 81% of the respondents offered placements in secure environments, with 19% not offering this opportunity. The placements ranged from three to sixteen weeks in length with a mean of 7.65 weeks.

The most common placement for students was in a Regional/Medium Secure Unit, with eighteen respondents utilising these placements. Intensive care units (9 respondents) and high dependency units (8 respondents) followed this. A number of prisons had been utilised for placements (six respondents) and a small number of respondents had placements in the high security Special Hospitals (six respondents). These latter figures may reflect the location of the educational establishments with those near to the Special Hospitals likely to make use of these facilities. The additional facilities identified by respondents included: a low secure unit, forensic services, admission/assessment unit, and a clinical therapies department. These additional facilities were only identified by single respondents and again may reflect the current development of services within a given locality. Given the current development of forensic services nationally it is likely that this configuration of placements could change considerably over the next three to five years. The expansion of community forensic services, low security units, increased medium secure unit beds, intensive care facilities and twenty four hour nursed beds becoming available (Department of Health 1998) will mean increased opportunity and scope for local practice placements.

Education providers were asked whether a placement in a secure environment was an optional or integral part of the pre-registration programme. The majority of respondents offer these placements on an optional basis to students (twelve respondents amounting to 44 per cent) with eight respondents (amounting to 29%) offering them as an integral part of the program. A small number of respondents (three; amounting to 11%) offered this as both an integral and optional part of the programme (it is presumed that there is a mandatory part of the programme with an option for the student at a later stage in the training to take a further placement).

Education providers were asked whether they had set learning outcomes in relation to theory and practice for nursing people in secure settings. The analysis of responses showed that ten (37 per cent) had objectives for neither theory nor practice. One respondent stated that they had outcomes for practice alone and a further six respondents (22 per cent) have learning outcomes for theory alone. Only ten of the respondents (37 per cent) had learning outcomes for both theory and practice for nursing people in secure settings.

When asked what should be a minimum requirement for inclusion in pre-registration programmes, participants in the focus groups and focused interviews varied greatly in their views on the range of input to the programme. This range included the view at one extreme, that there should be a Forensic Mental Health Branch ($n=1$), through to lectures from practitioners.

Findings (Pre-registration)

Mentally Disordered Offenders are in contact with a wide range of mental health services from community programmes and diversion schemes through to in-patient facilities in high secure hospitals. With this in mind there should be consideration given to increasing the knowledge and skills base in relation to MDOs within the Mental Health and Learning Disabilities Branch programmes.

During the course of the project it became clear that a general belief is held by registered nurses in secure services at all levels - pre-registration fails to meet the needs of the service. The Common Foundation programme is too long and too adult focused, and students frequently lack the practical, communication and inter-personal skills required for practice. Again these views are supported within the literature on the branch programmes generally. Eraut *et al.* (1995) and May *et al.* (1997) recommended that there was an increase in mental health and learning disability content within CFP and that counselling skills and stress management would benefit all students. The authors, May *et al.* (1997), McEvoy (1995) and the Sainsbury Centre for Mental Health (1997), also suggest that the length of the CFP should be altered to either a one year or a six month period.

Nursing in Secure Environments is a diverse concept, patients fit into all categories associated with branch programmes, i.e. Adult, Child, Mental Health and Learning Disabilities and are managed in a wide range of settings in the public and private sectors of health care and the Prison Services. There are many examples of good practice where attempts to enhance nursing provision and professional development are occurring, but from the work undertaken to date a number of recurring themes and concerns have emerged.

These themes and concerns are not only being voiced by practitioners and managers, but are also being raised by education providers. The methodologies that have been used, and the number of nurses contributing to the study validate the need for these issues to be addressed.

The main themes and concerns that are emerging from this work are as follows:

- time constraints and conflicting demands on pre-registration programmes both within the common foundation programme and the branch programmes
- availability and access to secure environments for placements
- lack of learning outcomes in relation to theory and practice
- apparent lack of knowledge and understanding amongst education staff about services for patients in secure environments
- lack of research activity by educational establishments in relation to secure nursing care
- disparity of views as to whether this topic should be included in pre-registration or post registration education programmes
- students emerge from pre-registration programmes without the appropriate competencies to undertake the role of a registered practitioner
- service needs and cost constraints preclude effective preceptorship for newly qualified nurses

To address these issues and to provide guidance and support to nurses in secure environments a number of agencies and entities need to be involved. These include the National Boards for Nursing, Midwifery and Health Visiting, Education Commissioning Consortia, Educational Institutions, service providers within Health and the Prison Services both in the public and private sectors and staff side organisations. The Future Organisation of Prison Health Care report urges the UKCC and other professional Royal Colleges, to bring nurses and doctors into contact with prison care during their period of training, and to broaden the knowledge and understanding of prison medicine and nursing.

Post Registration and Continuing Professional Development

Participants in the Scoping Exercise suggest that in order to meet the needs of the client groups, different skill bases are required for nurses working in each sector. Nurses in prison settings need to have skills and knowledge that transcend parts of the register, i.e. RGNs need to have some knowledge of Mental Health and Learning Disabilities and vice versa. Nurses in health care settings need competencies that may also be relevant to nurses in general psychiatric settings, but they may need to be more finely honed and have a different knowledge base because of the client group, the risk they present and the security needs of the service.

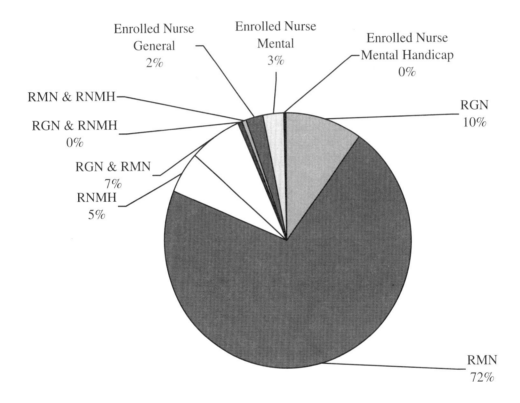

Figure 4.4.1 Registered Qualifications within the Health Sector

From the charts it is evident that the majority of nurses in the Prison Services have a General Qualification as opposed to hospitals were RMNs are pre-dominant. This pattern of qualifications does not appear to reflect the current needs of the prison population, an issue that has also been identified by the Prison Inspectorate who report that "In the majority of the establishments we looked at, the expertise of the staff, whilst excellent, was not specific to caring for patients in custody. One major problem is that different types of prisons need distinct skills from their staff." (HM Inspectorate of Prisons 1998)

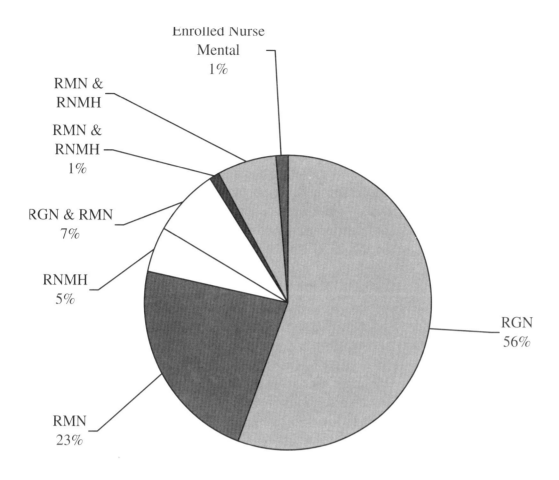

Figure 4.4.2. Registered Qualifications within Prison Settings

Although the data gathered shows that there is a major investment in education and training, both in the Prison Services and the health sector, an analysis of the responses from 714 staff questionnaires indicates that over 60% of nurses in both sectors do not have post registration qualifications. This is indicated below.

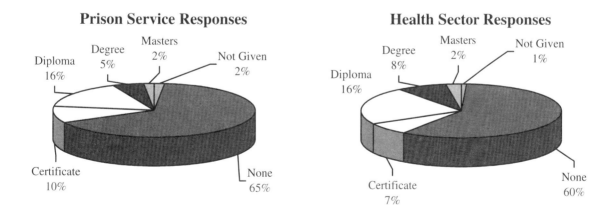

Figure 4.4.3 Post Registration Qualifications

95

A wide range of programmes are available to nurses in these areas, including academic programmes at a range of levels together with skills based programmes designed to meet organisational and individual need. However, access is a problem that many nurses have encountered. Either providers are not meeting local needs, or nurses have problems in having time off because of work pressures.

The opportunities for nurses to undertake further education and training following registration are wide and varied. The sample showed that the number of education and training days undertaken by nurses over the last twelve months ranges from 0 to 186 (one year full time education programme) with the mean being 10.57 (SD=16.95, min=0, max=186)days for Nurses working in prison and 15.85 (SD= 21.19, min=0, max=186)days for health service nurses, almost an average of 50% more. This mean difference is very highly significant (p <0.001).

Many nurses also believe that the majority of training and development opportunities are focused around formal organised courses and that a greater emphasis should be given to shadowing, secondments, conference attendance, project work and visits. Within the Prison Services a significant number of nurses mentioned that the study leave they undertook focused primarily on mandatory training rather than continuing professional development related to their nursing role. This issue is common in both sectors, and is supported by the recent study by Robinson and Kettles (1998) which reported that "training and education is patchy and poorly done", and the report by the Joint and NHS Executive working Group "The Future Organisation of Prison Health Care (1999) which states that "Arrangements for the continuing professional development of health care staff were not well established".

The majority of employers acknowledge the need and provide continuing professional development, covering a range of themes, in a variety of ways. (Refer Tables 4.4.4 and 4.4.5)

Figure 4.4.4 Do you have education or training programmes to prepare staff for working in a secure environment?

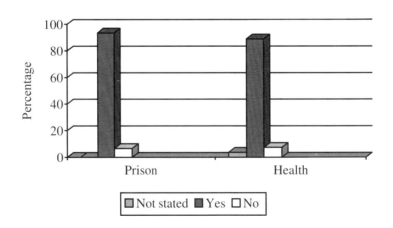

Figure 4.4.5 Types of education and training provided by the employer

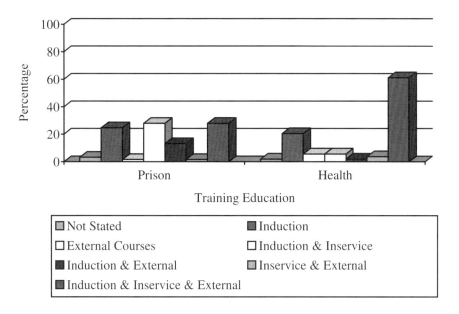

Although the education and training events potentially available to nurses is wide and varied, many staff expressed the view that the biggest deficit is their ability to attend events. Staff often reported that they are working on minimum numbers and unable to be given time off to participate in education and training. Some nurses do participate in their own time, although many reported the lack of opportunity to take their time back.

Figure 4.4.6 Source of education and training provision

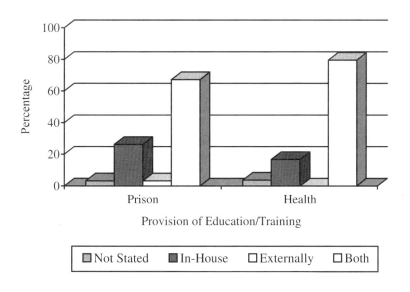

Education provision within Higher Education

Educational providers were asked to provide details of national board and other courses that they felt were relevant to nursing in secure environments. Table 4.4.1 and Table 4.4.2 provide the detail of these responses.

Table 4.4.1   Courses offered, seen as being relevant to nurses in secure environments

Course Name	N	% of those which offer
Control and Restraint techniques – Training for Trainers	4	10.4
Preventing and Managing Violence and Aggression	4	10.4
Recognition and Management of Substance Abuse	3	7.8
Teaching and Assessing in Clinical Practice	3	7.8
Principles of Psychiatric Nursing in Secure Environments	2	5.2
Risk Assessment/Management	2	5.2
Psycho-social Interventions	2	5.2
Mental Health and People with learning disabilities	2	5.2
Child and Adolescent Mental Health	1	2.6
Enhanced Practice in Mental Health	1	2.6
Care of the Mentally Disordered Offender	1	2.6
Coping with Violence and Aggression	1	2.6
Coping with Violence and Aggression	1	2.6
Care and Management of people in need of intensive mental health care	1	2.6
Nursing within Controlled Environments	1	2.6
Care of the Mentally Disordered Offender: Principles and Practice	1	2.6
Cognitive Behaviour Therapy	1	2.6
Acute Psychiatric Nursing	1	2.6
Social Learning Theory and Practice in Applied Settings	1	2.6
Working with people who have serious mental health problems and their families	1	2.6
Developments in Psychiatric Nursing	1	2.6
Recognition and Management of Substance Abuse	1	2.6
Care of People with AIDS and HIV related conditions	1	2.6
Caring for people with a dementing illness	1	2.6
Care of people with a mental illness/learning disability in community residential and day services	1	2.6
Counselling skills in caring relationships	1	2.6
Principles of health promotion and education for health	1	2.6
Principles of Child Protection	1	2.6
Understanding Research	1	2.6

Table 4.4.2 List of other perceived relevant courses cited by respondents

Course Title	N	% of those which offer
Forensic Mental Health Practice levels 2&3	4	10.4
Dip HE Forensic Psychiatric Nursing	3	7.8
Diploma /Degrees in Adult Mental Health	3	7.8
Specialist Practitioner	2	5.2
Prevention and Management of Suicide	2	5.2
Enhanced Practice in Mental Health Nursing	2	5.2
Clinical risk assessment	1	2.6
Post Grad MSc/ Higher award	1	2.6
Physical Intervention skills in managing violence	1	2.6
BSc Psycho-therapeutic interventions	1	2.6

Clinical Supervision, Preceptorship and Mentorship

The implementation of Clinical Supervision in practice is perceived by staff to be limited. There are some examples of effective clinical supervision although these are inconsistent both within and between units.

A number of nurses expressed a belief that clinical supervision is not particularly productive or valued and an optional part of their role. The purpose of clinical supervision is not accountability but Learning and Development. Clinical supervision has been described as "an interpersonal process within which the supervisor facilitates the development of the supervisee. The purpose is the development of the supervisee's abilities so that he/she returns to the client with greater consciousness. The primary aim of clinical supervision is learning and development, not accountability. As soon as accountability is introduced into the system the potential for learning and development is reduced." (Consedine 1998)

Many staff understand the concepts of clinical supervision, but the responses from the staff questionnaires indicate that a significant number are not aware of the guidance provided by UKCC on this issue. Only 45% of the 420 responses from the Prison Services had read the UKCC guidance compared with 87% from a sample of 240 hospital nurses.

Many nurses believe that clinical supervision is not a part of their employing organisation's culture and therefore not as valued as it could be. It is interesting to note that from the responses received, education programmes relating to Clinical Supervision and Reflective Practice are not mentioned.

In the Prison Services this is a particular problem because of the structure and culture, the small numbers of nurses in the system, nurses frequently being managed by non-nurses and because of isolation from other nurses. The recommendation of the Prison Services and NHS Executive working group to link Prison Services Healthcare with the local NHS should result in "professional isolation of health care staff being minimised, implying availability of professional supervision, opportunity for career moves between prison and NHS, access to in-service training, informal professional networks and research" (HM Prison Service and NHS Executive 1999)

There are a small number of individuals participating in Mentorship schemes but these tend to be informal, and linked to induction, rather than as part of a personal development plan.

Preceptorship schemes also exist both as formal and informal systems in a minority of organisations. There is wide support that this should be formally developed and available to all newly qualified nurses or for those returning to practice.

Staff appraisal and personal development planning

Results from the audits and from focus groups confirmed that access to, and implementation of staff appraisal and personal development planning was not consistent. Although the Prison Services operates an annual system of personal reviews within the health care sector only a small number of nurses participate in any systematic and long-term objective setting. Some staff have participated in appraisal systems in the past but believe that these were not maintained for a variety of reasons. On the whole, most nurses perceive staff appraisal as a positive opportunity but feel that they require more information and guidance about it.

Nurses identified lack of succession planning as a current weakness and suggest that it may in part be the result of the absence of any clear individual aspirational and development plans.

Induction

Induction of staff into a new post or new role should be seen as an investment. The inductee should be confident that they are familiar with policies, protocols and working practices as soon as possible on commencement in the job. However, the induction process varies from organisation to organisation both within the Prison Services and health care. On one end of a continuum nurses receive a comprehensive on-going structured induction with appropriate mentorship, whilst at the other nurses undertake new roles with minimal preparation and are potentially being put at risk.

A review of the Prison Inspection Reports supports this view, "In most instances staff, when they had actually received it, felt the induction and/or training was insufficient" (HM Inspectorate of Prisons 1998). One example cited is of "newly appointed mental health nurses at ... Prison who were left "to sink or swim" because managers failed to set up proper induction programmes". This situation is less common within hospitals, but examples have been given where induction takes place up to two months after commencement in post. In Northern Ireland permanent staff previously received a nine week programme, this has been revised to a four week programme supported by a period of supernumerary supervision, and all agency nurses receive a three day programme followed by a period of "shadowing".

Another aspect of Induction that causes concern is in relation to nurses who are not directly employed by an organisation, who provide a specialist service or provide nursing on an ad hoc basis. This group includes agency and bank nurses, Midwives, Health Visitors and CPNs. A number of participants in the focus groups indicated that the preparation given to these nurses and midwives was less rigorous, or missing altogether.

Topics that were regularly suggested by participants in the Focus Groups for inclusion in Induction programmes included

- Physical Interventions (Control and Restraint (C and R)), including Breakaway techniques and de-escalation techniques
- Management of aggression
- "Jail Craft" (for nurses working in prison)
- Security training (for health service staff)
- Boundaries and relationships
- Custody versus Care
- Risk assessment and Risk Management
- Suicide Awareness
- Records and record keeping (appropriate to organisation)
- Organisational policies, procedures and protocols
- Medications in common usage
- Legislation
- Offending behaviour

The availability, length and content of Induction Programmes are inconsistent. The most effective induction programmes appear to be those where there is a period of time when the inductee is supernumerary, mentorship is in place and initial induction is to the organisation and secondary induction to the individual's workplace

Physical Interventions

A number of staff stressed the need for Control and Restraint or "C and R" this was interpreted as an assertion that training in some form of physical intervention skills was seen as a pre-requisite for practice in this area. Control and Restraint, in its original form was initially developed by the Prison Service in England in the early 1980s (Paterson and Leadbetter 1999). It became the first widespread systematic approach to the physical management of violence to be used by nurses in the UK when the Special Hospitals introduced the system in England, following tuition from the prison service. In some hospitals this has been adapted to a form of physical intervention called "Care and Responsibility" in an effort to move away from what some have interpreted as a punitive model. However both sectors use the abbreviation C and R regularly. The Scottish Prison Service Nursing Service have revised their approach to physical interventions and a strategy for implementation of this approach has been developed.

Paterson and Leadbetter (1999) suggest that a degree of confusion has been allowed to develop around the exact inventory of techniques and the lack of and central regulatory mechanism. This has meant that a number of differing versions of "C and R" have ultimately developed, offered by a variety of organisations and individuals. Given the number of agencies offering restraint training, or incorporating elements in various modified forms it is not possible, at this point to regard the term "C and R" as a unitary entity in a national context and the extent of variation is a source of concern. These concerns are borne out in the scoping exercise.

Access to the appropriate training, and confusion about the level of involvement in Physical Restraint processes are the main issues confronting nurses. The issue has been of concern to nurses in other areas of nursing care, and the Institute of Psychiatry has undertaken research in 1998. The Psychiatric Nursing Section of the Institute carried out a survey to, describe the types of control and restraint training provided in hospitals in England and Wales, including the variety of techniques taught, and of training providers who offer such courses. The survey also sought to ascertain whether the practice of control and restraint matched Trust policies, and to describe the subjective experiences of nurses involved in the application of control and restraint techniques.

The survey obtained 294 responses, of which 46% were from females and 54% from males. The highest number of responses (n=104, 37%) were from staff nurses. 80% of the sample had a professional nursing qualification. Only 39% of respondents received C&R training in the first 3 months after starting work on their ward. 13% of respondents waited more than 2 years for training. 41% of respondents did not know to which organisation their instructor belonged. Training varied in duration from 5 - 21 days. The technique most frequently taught was verbal de-escalation, followed by restraint using a 3 person team, and the third most frequently taught technique was for taking the patient to the ground

Questions about the last incident in which the respondent was involved in C&R showed that in 19% of cases staff were injured, and in 11% of cases patients were injured (n=33). After the incident only 61% of respondents were de-briefed, and 76% were given documentation for audit procedures. About half of respondents (55%) had post-incident discussion review with the patient. This survey confirms findings from the focus groups and audits conducted across the UK in both the health sector and the Prison Services, in relation to debriefing and post incident discussions..

Findings (Post registration)

The Future Organisation of Prison Health Care report has identified that action needs to be taken to develop a strategy for the continuing professional development of health care professionals working in prisons. The report also suggests that the prison health care service is isolated from the mainstream of NHS development and that the current training and development of health care professionals is patchy. From the data captured during this scoping exercise a similar conclusion can be reached about some aspects of education and training of nurses in secure hospital provision.

The main issues that emerged from the study, which are common to both sectors, are in relation to:

• Clinical Supervision
• Induction
• Physical Intervention (Control & Restraint (C and R) training)

As previously stated, Clinical Supervision is sparse in implementation and a significant number of nurses are not aware of the guidance provided by the UKCC on this issue. In the Prison Services there is some uncertainty about whether clinical supervision should be provided by Prison Services nurses or by nurses within the local NHS. The general blockage to the implementation of Clinical Supervision appears to be lack of resources both in terms of time and expertise of nurses to provide this service to colleagues.

Induction needs to be more structured. The current variety in content, time available and mentorship has the potential to put nurses and their colleagues at risk. There were a significant number of examples provided during the focus groups, focused interviews and audits to support this concern. There is a general consensus that a supernumerary, modular, competence based, validated induction programme would be attractive and beneficial to nurses in both sectors. There are a number of common needs that have been identified as well as organisation or individual specific needs, therefore a modular programme could be developed which would acknowledge previous experience and allow practitioners to develop an appropriate, tailored programme.

"Control and Restraint" is an issue of concern across both sectors. Nurses have articulated the need to develop national standards for physical interventions when there is a breakdown in relationships that result in physical aggression. Linked to this nurses need to be conversant with the skills and knowledge to identify risk factors and de-escalation techniques.

Whatever approach is taken it is apparent that standardisation across each sector is essential. We have encountered a number of approaches that have been taken to prepare nurses in this area but in some instances nurses have been placed at risk because the preparation is inadequate, inappropriate or too long after commencing in the role. This issue is contentious because the different sectors have differing needs and the roles and responsibilities of nurses vary, also for some organisations C and R training generates significant income.

Employers need to consider their expectation of nurses, and the findings from the Institute of Psychiatry survey could be used to address the issues identified. The key findings were: staff are not always trained promptly and there is no clear policy about refresher courses; staff often do not know who trained their trainers, or who employs them, which can cause problems of accountability; the meaning of "control and restraint" varies widely and there is great variation in the duration of training; the content of courses may have inadequate coverage of the theoretical, preventative and defensive aspects of managing violence and aggression and nurses' responsibility for patient safety and dignity may not be given sufficient emphasis. Consequently, staff may lack confidence in their ability to use control and restraint techniques, which increases the risk of injury to both patients and staff. Post-incident debriefing, which should happen in all cases, does not occurring about a quarter of cases.

Conclusions

Educationalists, key informants in organisations and practitioners themselves were asked for both qualitative and quantitative information about their preparation , induction and ongoing professional development for working in secure care.

Pre-registration

- There are considerable time constraints and conflicting demands on pre-registration programmes both within the common foundation programme and the branch programmes in relation to experience within secure environments

- There is a low availability and access to secure environments for placements

- There is a lack of specific learning outcomes in relation to theory and practice for placements in secure environments

- There is a perception that education staff have a lack of knowledge and understanding about services for patients in secure environments

- There is limited research activity by educational establishments in relation to nursing practice in secure environments

- There is a disparity of views as to whether this topic should be included in pre-registration or post registration education programmes

- Students may emerge from pre-registration programmes with limited competencies to undertake the role of a registered practitioner in a secure environment

- Service needs, and a reported lack of resources, preclude effective preceptorship for newly qualified nurses. Students need support and leadership in these placements

Post Registration

- A strategic approach appears to be lacking in some areas in the development of the workforce to meet patient and organisational need.

- It appears that way in which individuals are supported in their continuing professional development is ad hoc, in that some individual practitioners receive a significant investment in development whilst others receive little or none..

- There are a wide range of validated courses already available to those working in secure care and the Prison Services.

- There is limited evidence to state whether any post–reg courses improve competency for working in secure environments, the only examples cited of competence being enhanced were in relation to the "Thorn", Cognitive Behaviour Therapies and Psycho-Social Interventions programmes

Clinical Supervision

- There is a low level of acceptance of clinical supervision, possibly because practical problems and lack of management support create difficulties in its implementation which compounds the isolation of practitioners in circumstances which often test their professional resilience

- Clinical Supervision is not readily available to nurses who are working in conditions that test their professional resilience. The patient groups and professional isolation, in some instances, would suggest that this is an area where nurses would benefit from the rigorous application of Clinical Supervision.

- Systems of either formal or informal mentorship and preceptorship are not widely used.

Induction

- There appears to be a good understanding of what is necessary to correctly and properly induct nurses to work in secure environments. However, these are poorly implemented, do not follow a common pattern, and are not always scheduled to be available when new practitioners need them most.

- Effective induction could prevent some of the problems experienced and set the tone and culture of the organisation.

Physical Interventions

- The level of training and the physical and other interventions that nurses are expected to use, in the management of challenging behaviours, are unclear.

- National professional standards in physical interventions do not exist to guide nurses in the United Kingdom. Therefore there is no consistent application of standards when physical intervention is required

- The providers of programmes on physical intervention are not accredited and the content and modes of delivery vary considerably.

- Concerns have been expressed about the availability of training in physical interventions which potentially puts nurses at risk.

4.5 Identify issues faced in working with a client group who may compromise therapeutic nurse patient relationships, particularly with reference to personality disordered patients

Although the nurses involved in the Focus Groups and interviews identified people with a severe personality disorder as patients who potentially compromised relationships other patient groups were also identified. These included substance abusers, people with co-occurring disorders, people who self harm and women.

The concept of nurses behaving in particular ways as a consequence of feelings and attitudes towards individual and specific groups of patients is not a new phenomenon. The seminal work of Stockwell (1972) introduced the concept of "the unpopular patient" in her study of interpersonal relationships in general wards.

The original impetus for this study came from an interest in the care given to patients classified as "difficult" by the nursing staff, and from a need to know more about the problems presented by such patients in order to help nurses understand and care for them.

The study devised means of identifying popular and unpopular patients, explored possible reasons for patients being thus classified and examined the nurses' attitudes and behaviour towards them.

The chief aim of Stockwell's study was to determine whether there were some patients whom the nursing team enjoyed caring for more than others. If this proved to be so, to ascertain whether there was any measurable difference in the nursing care afforded to the most and least popular patients.

Reasons for patients' unpopularity were mostly related to "personality factors and physical defects such as deafness, but patients of foreign nationality and those whose present stay in hospital was longer than three months also proved to be significantly more unpopular than others." (Stockwell 1972)

Patients in Secure Environments

Studies have repeatedly shown that a high percentage of any forensic population can be expected to fulfil formal diagnostic criteria for one or more personality disorders. (Gunn *et al.* 1991, Maden *et al.* 1995).

Regardless of patients' formal psychiatric diagnoses, shared psychopathological characteristics exist amongst the population detained in hospital secure environments, which require a consistent response from the health care professionals managing this group. Milieu therapy has been highlighted as a potential approach with some success in personality disordered populations (Dolan and Coid 1993) but has been criticised in its application in secure environments (Fallon 1999), particularly so from nursing with its primary base within the social environment. The feelings, attitudes and behaviour of nurses risk being compromised by the very nature of interpersonal transactions that are part of their role.

Complications which arise when the organisation as a whole fails to create systems of care which take into account the patients' psychopathologies are clear (Fallon 1999). Examples of harrowing, disabling incidents and untoward events which are traumatic for the nursing discipline as a whole, have characterised the care for this group in recent years as evidenced in a number of public enquiries (Department of Health 1992, Department of Health 1999).

There seems little guidance available to adequately prepare nurses for the task of carrying out long term care within secure services where the patients' criminality is as much a part of the psychopathological picture as the psychiatric diagnosis. Based on the premise that personality disorders, especially antisocial and borderline are likely to predominate amongst patients detained in forensic services whether there are other co existing mental disorders or not, it would seem that the primary concern for nursing should be a theoretical framework for forensic patients in general. This should be informed by the factors that mediate risk, diagnoses and offending rather than diagnoses alone. (Aiyegbusi 1997)

Personality Disorder

In the last ten years, interest in Personality Disorder research has shown substantial growth. Research interest in Personality Disorders is indicated by the fact that over 750 empirical studies are abstracted in the American Psychological Association Psyche-lit database, covering the five year period of January 1987 to June 1992. The Journal of Personality Disorders is devoted exclusively to this area. The many national and international conferences and workshops that have been held on Personality Disorders are testament to its growth.

This large and growing literature on Personality Disorders should not obscure the fact that there are serious theoretical and methodological problems with the whole enterprise of diagnosing Personality Disorder. Indeed, the last rigorous evaluation of the diagnosis and treatment efficacy for this patient group carried out by one of the Reed subgroups in 1992. Dolan and Coid (1993) outlined the major problems and disagreements amongst clinicians about the diagnosis of this condition and, if diagnosis was agreed, whether in fact the condition was amenable to treatment.

The issue of Personality Disorder was the area of most commentary, from participants in the scoping exercise, in relation to a patient group that they felt presented the most severe and sustained problems in both the criminal justice and secure health care system. This has been a topic of much heated debate in recent times, it is an issue that is being addressed by the NHS Executive as identified in the recent Modernising Mental Health Services (NHS Executive 1998). It has been the subject of a two year judicial inquiry which reported in January 1999 (Fallon 1999) and made a number of key recommendations to the Government regarding the future care and management of the group(s) including changes to the legal system.

An analysis of the report provides the following observations:

Diagnosis requires observation over time because lying and conning may temporarily conceal the extent of disorder. The surveys of prison populations carried out in various studies in the United States and this country report prevalence rates of 11 per cent (Gunn 1999). It is suggested that a distinction needs to be made between a diagnosis for psychiatric purposes and a diagnosis that is going to lead to detention under secure conditions. It is also suggested that the legal criteria of serious anti-social behaviour and dangerous behaviour are a more reliable indicator to decide the need for security. The two indicators are somewhat different and certainly there are many more people who need help than there are who need detention. The law recognises this to a certain degree by having the system of restriction orders for more dangerous individuals.

There is an overlap between other psychiatric disorders and psychopathy insofar as, for example, those who are diagnosed as being of psychopathic personality are very much more likely than others to have areas of acute psychotic disturbance (Blackburn 1993). One of the problems is that the acute psychotic disturbances are readily diagnosed and assessed in the course of admission to hospital, but that when that condition subsides they tend to be discharged with the underlying personality disorder remaining and continuing to cause social problems.

In 1992 Dr Rosemary Cope carried out a survey of forensic psychiatrists, with a 95 per cent return rate, and almost 40 per cent of the respondents were "unenthusiastic" about the treatment of Personality Disorder. Another dilemma amongst health care professionals and the public is the debate about whether Personality Disorder even exists as a health deficit or is simply a social construct possibly akin to the biblical notion of evil.

The Fallon Inquiry team put forward the view that the main concern of the public is dangerousness. Therefore, there is an expectation that people with a personality disorder who offend should be dealt with as dangerous people, given whatever sentence is appropriate, perhaps renewing it under some new legislation, but only transferred to a therapeutic setting from prison if they were assessed and agreed that they would be likely to benefit.

Therapeutic Communities have been suggested as a method of managing and treating people with a Personality Disorder. The basis for a successful therapeutic community with a personality disordered patient has to be effectively a contract of care with the patient co-operating in a programme of treatment and care that is consistent and coherent (Storey and Dale 1998).

A new emphasis on evidence-based care and clinical effectiveness has become a priority within the NHS, and has highlighted specific issues in working with this group. Implementing evidence-based health care is particularly difficult given the debate as to the existence of personality disorder as a health deficit and ambiguity as to whether we are trying to treat the whole personality or just the offending behaviours. The final dilemma arises from the lack of research evidence as to which treatments are most effective.

Professor Don Grubin of Newcastle University compiled a "taxonomy of interventions" related to Personality Disorders. This ranged from what he considered to be the sublime to the ridiculous with treatment options such as psychodynamic psychotherapy or cognitive analytical psychotherapy standing alongside foot massage, horse riding and aromatherapy.(Grubin 1993)

What was particularly important from this research, however, was that Professor Grubin demonstrated that whilst we might have our own opinions as to which treatments are most effective with this group of patients, there is no tangible evidence demonstrating effectively which treatments work with which disorders or components of disorder related to personality. In effect we have to question whether psychotherapies are any more or less effective in the treatment of personality disorders than complimentary therapies.

In effect, nurses in forensic and Prison Services are charged with providing care for a large group of individuals with particularly challenging behaviours but whose disorders are nebulous and ill defined, whose treatment is often haphazard and whose outcomes in terms of clinical targets are poorly understood and progress difficult to measure.

Whilst the notion of Personality Disorder as a health deficit remains somewhat nebulous, it is recognised that the demonstrable factors indicating a diagnosis of Personality Disorder are most apparent through the manner in which an individual perceives, interprets and relates to his environment and others (Melia 1997). In acknowledging this and trying to provide a treatment service for this group of individuals it is apparent that "relationship" has to be the one significant key pathway towards appropriate clinical treatment. People with a Severe Personality Disorder demonstrate emotional extremes of love and hate and levels of anger and hostility are particularly high and are most commonly focused towards those on whom individuals are most reliant, in effect the staff (Melia 1997).

In relating to others, such individuals demonstrate an expectation that they will be harmed, exploited and let down and they will enter into relationships with this expectation in mind. They will often demonstrate an exaggerated moral outrage if they feel their own personal rights or wants have been violated, but will disregard the rights of others, demonstrating no remorse for having wronged another and showing no capacity to experience guilt or to profit from experience, often to the point were they will feel justified in having hurt or mistreated others. Staff working within this environment may be exposed to such social dynamics for extensive periods of time and for all of their working days.

In this environment, then, the issue of boundaries in inter-personal relationships is fundamental to the therapeutic process, both for the protection of the staff member and to aid the progress of the patient.

Melia (1997) describes two main themes that need to be managed by nurses when dealing with this group of patients, these are relationships and splitting and secrets.

At the outset, the relationship between the patient and his clinical team members is relatively neutral with clear boundaries dictated by professional standards and cultural expectation. The process of assessment and treatment, however, can challenge the social construct of a neutral relationship, as the discussion will often relate to the most intimate and intrusive components of the patient's life, experience and feelings. This can be particularly difficult for the nurse who will spend long periods of time with the patients in community settings and through a range of private and public experiences. Gutheil *et al.* note three degrees or levels of challenge to relationship boundaries, namely "boundary crossing, boundary violation and sexual misconduct," They further note that the care environment can predict the violation of boundaries and that "various group therapeutic approaches or therapeutic communities may involve inherent boundary violations."

In forensic services this is complicated by the nature of offending behaviours that has led individuals to be admitted.

Splitting is a process of making an individual or group feel different (normally better or worse) than their peers or those around them. In practice the negative splitting behaviours are often quickly picked up; for example a patient may claim a specific staff (or staff group) is victimising him by not facilitating a request that he claims others do (even if this is contrary to the ward/hospital policies). In this the patient is both exerting a pressure on the member of staff who is attempting to maintain consistent practice to alter or 'bend' the rules thereby creating conflict between staff members.

More destructive than this, however, are the seductive components to splitting which are more easily missed and can have a greater effect; for example when the patient invests an apparent trust and confidence in a particular member of the care team. This is further complicated and distorted when the patient invites the team member to maintain 'secrets' often in the name of confidentiality. This can be particularly divisive when more than one discipline is involved and can lead to major conflicts amongst the clinical care team. (Melia 1997)

Dale *et al* (1999) suggests that forensic patients often bring to their relationship, with any worker, high levels of emotional need and vulnerability and the experience of abuse and manipulation. Previous dysfunctional relationships add to the proclivity to distort and misinterpret the behaviour and signals given out by others. Most offenders are prepared to trust and reveal personal feelings and experiences, in this context, but may expect an equal investment on the part of the worker.

Boundaries within professional practice are used to define acceptable conduct and limits of practice. Much of the writing, particularly within the psychotherapy literature, has focused upon the area of sexual misconduct, this being an extreme example that identifies the relationship complexities in mental health care.

It is easy to see the potential for role boundaries to break down should the worker lose focus and concentration, when daily walking the tightrope of care and control. Staff need to have clearly defined professional boundaries between themselves and their patients. Development and maintenance of these boundaries is the shared responsibility of the individual staff member, their line manager and their colleagues within the multi-disciplinary team.

Epstein and Simon (1990) describe other areas where boundary violation and exploitation can occur. These include excessive familiarity; dependency; non-clinical business dealings and breaches of confidentiality. In a recent Canadian study of nurses views on professional boundaries (Gallop 1997) the nurse participants were in agreement about a taboo on sexual contact but less clear on other boundaries. Pillette *et al.* (1995) assert that role definitions assign to the nurse the responsibility of "separating and containing his/her needs separately from the patients needs".

Gallop (1997) suggests that professionals contemplating the appropriateness of various activities should ask themselves "would I do/say this in front of my supervisor, would I tell my supervisor/colleague what I have done/said- if not why not?" Secrecy is usually a central tenet of boundary violation and often starts with a small slip, such as excessive self-disclosure, and proceeds on to a special relationship that may include secrecy.

Gutheil and Gabbard (1993) point out clinicians should be aware of three principles that govern relationships: boundary crossings, boundary violations (a harmful crossing) and sexual misconduct. Boundaries for these purposes cover the following:

1. Role
2. Time
3. Place and space
4. Money, gifts, services and related matters
5. Clothing
6. Language
7. Self-disclosure
8. Physical contact

Mental Health care is based on the establishment of a therapeutic relationship. Institutional life, particularly in the long term settings of many forensic services, may mean that nursing staff are placed in situations that test boundaries or provide a degree of informality that threatens the necessary therapeutic endeavour.

The therapeutic relationship is the primary intervention for the nurse and is founded upon a basis of trust, respect and the appropriate use of power. Boundaries within the treatment setting must be clear and not transgressed. To do otherwise creates an ambiguous, confusing and possibly frightening environment for patients and staff. On these issues psychiatric nursing texts are clear: do not get over involved; don't have secrets from the team; seek out consultation or supervision. (Dale *et al.* 1999)

Substance Abuse

Co-occurring disorders are used to describe the individuals who have a DSM IV Axis 1 major mental disorder (e.g. psychotic, depressive, and bipolar disorders) and a substance use disorder.

Given the increasing incidence of mentally ill and/or substance abusing individuals who are seen in courts, community settings and prisons, greater attention has been given to the need for diversion and rehabilitation programmes in these settings. These reflect a need to develop specialised treatment interventions for mentally disordered and substance-abusing offenders.

The presence of co-occurring mental health and substance abuse disorders generally indicate a poor prognosis for involvement in treatment (McLellan 1986, Weiss 1992) and compliance with medication (Drake *et al.* 1989), and is associated with greater rates of hospitalisation (Safer 1987), more frequent suicidal behaviour (Caton 1981), and difficulties in social functioning (Evans and Sullivan 1990).

Accurate assessment of co-existing disorders also presents difficult challenges, due to the residual affects of addictive substances (e.g. withdrawal effects) that may mask or mimic psychiatric symptoms such as depression. Dually diagnosed individuals may also present acute psychiatric symptoms such as anxiety and depression that may interfere with traditional forms of substance abuse treatment, and more often require hospitalisation or participation in intensive mental health services (Evans and Sullivan 1990; Pensker 1983). Involvement and retention of offenders with co-occurring disorders in treatment is often difficult, due to rationalisation and blaming others for their difficulties, distrust of service providers, and sudden changes in psychiatric symptoms.

A potential barrier in accessing services for this population is the absence of co-ordinated mental health and substance abuse services in prisons and in community settings. This is often due to lack of awareness, confidentiality issues, and waiting lists for treatment services. In the USA dually diagnosed offenders are frequently excluded from some community treatment programmes due to severe mental health and substance abuse problems, use of psychiatric medication and to their criminal justice history. (Peters and Hills 1993)

The research literature has shown that individuals with co-occurring disorders experience considerable fluctuations in their motivation and commitment to behaviour change during the early phases of treatment. Despite their attendance and treatment, offenders are not often initially committed to the idea of becoming abstinent (Drake *et al.* 1996), and require ongoing work to promote motivation. If unaddressed these issues are likely to lead to high rates of dropout and non-adherence to treatment regimes.

In the absence of comprehensive and integrated services, these individuals tend to repeatedly cycle through treatment, probation and prison, and are at higher risk for substance abuse relapse and other behaviours that often lead to more involvement with the criminal justice system. Offenders with co-occurring disorders are more likely to re-offend or to receive sanctions when they are not taking medication, when they are not in treatment, and when they are experiencing mental health symptoms.

Offenders with co-occurring disorders are more likely to have cognitive limitations that affect their supervision, such as difficulties in attention and concentration, memory, abstract reasoning, problem solving, and planning ability.

Women's Issues

Although female patients make up less than one fifth of the population in secure settings in Britain (Hemmingway 1996), as a group they are a "heterogeneous collection of women with a wide range of ages, personal, psychiatric and forensic histories, who nevertheless share some characteristics and experiences" (Dolan and Bland 1996). However, women patients are also different from male patients in significant ways: women patients are less likely to have committed serious criminal offences in comparison with men, but are more likely to have experienced previous psychiatric admission (Bartlett 1993). WISH (1999) report that the current secure provision does not meet women's security needs, they require high intensive care, with a high staff/patient ratio, providing a supportive and safe environment rather than physical high security care.

A higher proportion of women than men in high security care in England and Wales have arrived there from within the NHS psychiatric services as a result of being regarded as difficult to manage within lower levels of security. (Lart *et al.* 1998) Women in high secure settings are more likely to be admitted because of damage to property, suicidal or self-harming behaviour or as the result of aggressive behaviour towards staff in psychiatric hospitals of lesser security. (WISH 1999)

When compared with men in secure environments, women are more likely to present a risk of violence to current caregivers or fellow patients than to the general public. Risk of harm to self is also high (Leibling 1997, WISH 1999). This is likely to be increased by regression associated with detention in a secure environment where fellow patients and caregivers replicate family dynamics (Travers and Aiyegbusi 1998). In the midst of a number of internal and external risk factors, active psychosis seems to be the single most important mediator of risk to others. The more psychotic, the more dangerous any individual patient is. Dissociation while simultaneously experiencing severe command hallucinations or terrifying flashbacks which can possibly be considered as extreme examples of numbing and intrusion, seem to feature among the most dangerous symptoms patients may experience (Travers and Aiyegbusi 1998). Risk of harm to self is also high (Leibling 1997, WISH 1999).

There is a high risk of splitting between those members of the team who work with these patients and other non-ward based professionals and family and friends. A common theme involves professionals, visitors or clinical staff, after being filled with projections about neglect and mistreatment, feeling that they have to do something to rescue the patient(s) from their situation. Current caregivers, already feeling persecuted and invalidated, become increasingly guarded and defended against perceived external threat to the point where scrutiny of any kind is experienced as severely invasive and punishing. All parties then fear collaborative working because of their anxieties about identifying with the "opposition." (Travers and Aiyegbusi 1998) It is only by working together in consistent, integrated teams that professionals can avoid splitting and attacking each other. The challenge is to provide a care and treatment service for patients but this is difficult when energy and resources are channelled into operating defensively. Defences tend to involve uncoordinated action rather than focused, considered thought and debate.

Adshead (1997) discusses how the patients' need for their fantasised, idealised caregiver leads to denigration of less than ideal care, which is perceived as abuse. Verbal, emotional and physical attacks on caregivers, which are usually forced to provide less than perfect care, are commonplace. Both Main (1957) and Menzies Lyth (1988) describe the agony experienced by caregivers when their attempts to "cure" are thwarted by patients who refuse to get better.

Travers and Aiyegbusi (1998) explain that much of these dynamic processes can be understood in terms of occurring through the transferences and countertransferences that operate within the wards and clinical areas. Rage toward past abusive and neglecting caregivers, which had been dissociated from, is now displaced onto current caregivers who are then emotionally perceived in the same way. As Head (1997) points out: "The clinical team may not be able to deal with the patient's feelings, but they can (and must) make an attempt to deal with their own."

Herman (1992) states that some of the most astute descriptions of traumatic transference can be found in the literature about clinical encounters involving individuals who are diagnosed with borderline personality disorder and were written before the traumatic roots of the disorder were known. Current diagnosis gives high figures for the presence of borderline personality disorder for both the secure health care and prison services for women.

Women with Borderline Personality Disorder find it difficult to cope in secure settings, in environments where they are surrounded by the distress of others and where they are controlled by disciplined regimes influenced by the custodial aspects of secure care, the affective vulnerability, lack of self-identity and sense of powerlessness experienced by women with BPD will be exaggerated. This is likely to promote increased impulsiveness including self-harming and assaultative behaviour. (WISH 1999)

Careful attention is required for the rigorous application of protective factors needed to ensure safety: these take the form of goals, rules, boundaries and support systems for caregivers (Herman 1992). In Women's Services, both within health care and the Prison Services, these protective factors need to be a key part of the working conditions for staff.

Self-harm in Secure Environments

The issue of self-harm, self-injury or mutilation, is one which is prevalent within secure environments in both the health care and criminal justice sectors. Within these two sectors there are differing numbers of self-harm incidents, but in the majority of cases the responses are the same.

One definition of self-harm is "deliberate damage to one's own body, irrespective of motivation and which required some form of intervention" (Swinton and Smith 1997). The main form of self-harming incidents are cutting, burning, swallowing and inserting foreign objects, both into wounds and orifices, overdosing on medication or ligature tying. Although many chronic self-harmers affirm that they have no intention to commit suicide and that they self-injure for a number of reasons quite unrelated to a desire to die it is often linked to suicide by the term parasuicide. Dolan (1998) suggests that the "majority of people who self-harm do not, in fact, go on to commit suicide", although the report from the National Confidential Inquiry into Suicide and Homicide by People with Mental Illness (Department of Health 1999) suggests that many do.

	92/93	93/94	94/95	95/96	96/97
Total no. of inmates self-harming	2,556	3,359	3,609	4,680	4,195
% of inmates self-harming per day	0.02%	0.02%	0.02%	0.02%	0.02%
Total no. of self-harm incidents	3,263	4,521	4,823	6,269	5,360
Female self-harm incidents	624	1,158	1,261	1,054	730
Adult men/YO male self-harm incidents	2,612	3,363	3,562	5,242	4,630

Table 4.5.1   Source: (Annual Report of HM Prison, Director of Health Care, England and Wales, 1996-97)

114

Although statistics from the Prison Services (Table 4.5.1) indicate that more men then women self-harm, the literature concentrates mainly on women's self-harming behaviour. This is because proportionally more women than men display this behaviour, for example, figures from 1995/6 show that out of 53,000 men, 5,242 self-harmed, 9.9%, whereas the figures for women show that from 2,300 inmates, there were 1,054 reported incidents of self harm. Statistics from a number of studies in prison show the following results - Morris and Rushton (1993) report 1/5 women self-harming, King (1994) reported a 24% incidence and Devlin 19 % (1998).

While the available statistics from mental health secure units are higher, the literature does not mention male self-harm incidences, Adshead (1994), reported that 80% of female patients in secure hospitals were suicidal or sought to self-harm. WISH (1999) suggests that women feel threatened in secure provision, particularly Medium Secure Units that are so male dominated. They go on to state that women will experience being physically restrained, being pinned down to be forcibly injected, often by male staff, as "legitimised" assaults against them. This exposure to harassment and abuse, and of feeling violation from staff are likely to be major contributing factors to their "unmanageable" behaviour and self harming.

Despite the high incidence of self-harming behaviour, and its possible severity, the literature reports an often negative response from staff. Liebling et al. found that "staff responses were perceived as unhelpful and punitive. The majority focused on self-harming behaviour and failed to address the underlying distress" (1997). In a study of women in prison, carried out by HM Chief Inspector of Prisons, it was discovered that "there is a tendency to respond to self-harm by incapacitation and the simplistic response of putting a women in isolation ... it might postpone the harm, but it does not deal with the cause" (1997).

Liebling et al. (1997) report typical staff comments were " 'you're causing too much paper work', 'attention seeker' and 'can't you see I'm busy'". In another study, staff reported that they "had been trained to deal with self-harm with control and restraint". It is felt that these responses are fuelled by a belief that the behaviour is used a tool of manipulation or attention seeking, and also as a "coping mechanism for staff who may feel in danger of being overwhelmed"(HM Chief Inspector of Prisons 1997). It should be noted here that it is not only nursing staff who responds in this way, but it is felt that "these attitudes may be more damaging because of the close daily contact between nurses and patients". (Liebling et al. 1997). These comments appear to show that the empathy felt by nurses is stretched, but that care needs are still met.

There is clear evidence that self-harming behaviour is often neither an attempt to manipulate or to gain attention, but rather a response to any number of deep-seated emotional problems. These can include previous sexual, physical and emotional abuse, regaining inner control, depression, anger and to reduce anxiety/tension. More importantly, self-harming behaviour is perceived by those who self-harm as a way of way of regaining control in lives which are epitomised by lack of control, often for the reasons outlined above. Bonnie Burstow explains, "control is a meaning that I have found to be absolutely invariable and the most fundamental. Women traditionally have been controlled by others and violated in ways which exceed the already devastating norm. Women who have felt the control acutely, desperately need some sense of power. They turn to the one area over which they have control, their own bodies" (Liebling *et al.* 1997). Given this view it is obvious the types of responses above will only serve to punish the women for their behaviour, and often can "reinforce aspects of power and control which served to exacerbate self-harming as one of the only ways women could continue to cope within a punishing environment" (Liebling *et al.* 1997).

If then these responses are inappropriate, what can be done in order to best help those with self-harming behaviour? Kelland in (HM Chief Inspector of Prisons 1997) says, "helping women prisoners who self-harm must involve listening to them, facilitating their understanding of why they self-harm and helping them to find alternative ways of coping".

The literature shows that often nurses are not adequately trained to deal with self-harm, and do not receive the necessary support when dealing with these incidents. Liebling *et al.* (1997) outlined the results from 83 staff responses with regard to support after they had discovered somebody who had self-harmed.

55   reported no formal support,
52   reported informal support from colleagues.
36   staff said they felt unsupported,
27   thought about the event constantly
27   felt the need to talk about the event constantly,
25   staff members felt dread, and
14   nurses had experienced nightmares as a result of the discovery.

Nurses in these environments are often criticised for the responses to self-harming behaviour outlined above, but as the literature shows they are often not supported after dealing with a traumatic events that they are not trained to properly understand or respond to. This is particularly disconcerting when it is discovered that these nurses are putting in requests for the training, but are often unable to access it due to lack of funding or the inability to get time off work. Liebling *et al.* 1997 outlines a number of questions they asked nurses, with regard to training, and they obtained the following results.

Have you received any training to deal with self-injury?
YES   **14%**   NO   **86%**

Would you benefit from further training?
YES   **91%**   NO   **9%**

Would you benefit from training on how to more effectively manage people who self-injure?
YES   **80%**   NO   **20%**

Would you benefit from training which gave you more knowledge about why people self-injure?
YES   **84%**   NO   **16%**

This suggests that the majority of these nurses feel they are inadequately prepared to deal with self-harming behaviour, and highlights many issues concerned with practice standards and professional responsibility. Greater emphasis needs to be paid to self-harming behaviour when preparing nurses to work in these environments, both for the benefit of the women and the staff. Dolan, (1998) suggests that "Prison staff need to be given the skills to act as counsellors, teachers and leaders, guiding self-harmers towards improving their own health. Perhaps more importantly we need to work towards an environment in which prisoners have ways open to them of expressing their feelings other than self-harm." This could help the self harmers to confront their behaviour, and try to find more positive ways of coping with their emotional problems, and aid the nurses facilitating this. Until such time as these issues are addressed, the never-ending cycle of self-harm is likely to continue, to the detriment of everybody involved.

Two courses have recently been launched looking specifically at the problem of self injury, one at Ashworth Hospital in Merseyside (commenced in 1998) and the other at Salford University (commenced in 1999) at academic levels 2 and 3 respectively. Both courses have significant contributions from users of services.

Findings

A detailed analysis has been conducted into the qualitative data generated from the focused interviews, focus groups and comments from the organisational questionnaire. It has been possible from this analysis to identify key themes which emerged as concerns for nursing staff in secure environments in both the Health and Criminal Justice sector these being diagnosis, substance abuse, suicide and self harm, emotional demands, management problems, cultural issues, complaints.

The groups of patients presenting the greatest difficulty for staff included patients with a personality disorder, mentioned by the majority staff, problems in relation to alcohol and drug abuse, women's issues (mainly linked the problem of borderline personality disorder) and self-harm, these findings support the literature on this subject area.

Diagnosis

The issues that face nurses in relation to the accurate diagnosis of patients is discussed in section 4.2

Substance Abuse

Nurses in the Prison Services identified the issue of detoxification of alcohol and drug abuse as a key problem which was not reflected within the health sector. It may be that health sector patients are generally received at a later stage following detention than in the criminal justice system and tend to see less chronic, persistent and heavy drug abusers.

Nursing staff reported that this was a group of patients where it was often difficult to distinguish between a need and a want, this was particularly so in relation to some demands for medication such as Benzodiazepines and opiate based analgesics. This group of patients is adept at putting staff under pressure and at targeting staff who they believe may be more sympathetic to their requests/demands. A particular concern and debate in the prison system is over the extending of prescribing rights to nurses in this sector. Whilst some anomalies exist with regard to in-possession and over the counter medications there could be clear advantages for patients if nursing staff had some prescribing rights extended to them, the consensus was that the disadvantages could outweigh the advantages. This was principally if it became known that this facility was available to them they would be placed under intense pressure from some patients to prescribe to them. If prescribing is to be considered, or extended, then explicit protocols, developed in conjunction with managers and pharmacists, need to be in place.

Suicide and Self Harm

Treatment issues in relation to self-harm and suicide were identified from both the Health and Prison sector, particularly so from the latter. Of some concern was a lack of consistency between and within services in relation to the existence of policies and the level of understanding of policies by the nursing staff. In Scotland the Prison Service have developed a suicide risk management strategy, "Act and Care", which provides all Scottish prison staff with a model within which to work. We also note with interest the recent work by the Standing Nursing and Midwifery Advisory Committee (SNMAC) who conducted some research into special observation policies in Mental Health services in the NHS. In this report they state, "Research on the nursing practice of observing patients who are at risk from self- harm, or of causing harm to others, shows that there is no consistency in the definition of terms, principles or processes. In some trusts there is no written policy for observation. Trusts vary greatly in the indications for observation and in the personnel that are thought appropriate to perform it. Where policies and procedures do meet a reasonable standard, they may not be implemented properly." (SNMAC 1999)

"Although some incidents of suicide or serious self- harm might not occur if nurses skills in assessment and observation were improved, the job of the nurse is often made more difficult by the architecture of in-patient units. Some serious incidents might be avoided if environmental dangers in in-patient wards were corrected. These include design faults, which prevent nurses from observing patients properly, or windows, particularly in upper floor wards, that they are unsuitably glazed" (SNMAC1999)

The findings from the secure environment project support these findings. Observations and feedback from nurses illustrated many instances of architectural and design problems. This was particularly true of the often outmoded and outdated building stock of the prison system as well as some newer and poorly designed secure environment in the health sector. Indeed, some designated secure environments in the health sector were secure in name only and in one instance had been purposely built to care for the elderly and the only alteration to accommodate mentally disordered offenders was the fitting of new locks on the doors.

Emotional Demands

It was clear when discussing difficult patients with nursing staff in secure environments that this group above all generate a great deal of emotion. The type of language the nurses used when discussing this group of people can exemplify this. Words regularly occurring included abuse, aggression, challenging, compromises, dangerous, difficult, manipulate, pressure, splitting, violence, vulnerability and problems. As can be seen from this daunting list of words, the nurses in close proximity to people who generate such intense feelings can be drawn into a dynamic whereby mistakes are made, demands are acceded to and boundaries crossed which in a less secure and intense atmosphere or environment might be easier to resist.

This range of patients undoubtedly has the capacity to disrupt services and emotionally engage staff. Given the demands and complexity of this group of people it was both surprising and alarming that clinical supervision of the staff was not routinely available and often staff were left to their own devices in relation to dealing with individuals and the emotions generated by them. This was particularly a feature of the Prison Services where nurses are not always managed by nurses.

Management Problems

Another key theme emerged in relation to the management problems of attempting to cope with these difficult patients on a day-to-day basis. Many examples were given whereby individuals had totally disrupted wards and departments to a stage where they became all but dysfunctional for periods of time. These patients can be an enormous strain upon resources particularly in relation to procedures such as special observations. An extreme example identified was an individual who required six nursing staff to be present at all times because of his risk of suicide but owing to his physical power required a large presence of nursing staff to respond to his needs. The situation persisted for several months and the final cost to the organisation was in excess of £300,000.

Maintenance of boundaries was identified as a key problem by a high percentage of nursing staff but only within the health sector; in the prison system is was not identified as a key problem. This may reflect the heavy reliance on physical security within the Prison Services. Even given the availability of high levels of physical security and sanction it is a matter of concern that these are the very group of patients were psychologically boundaries are most necessary to keep the patient and staff safe in carrying out nursing interventions. There was also a much lower level of knowledge and understanding of psychological processes relevant to managing violent incidents, which may reflect the more general nurse-orientated background of the prison system. In considering education and training needs for staff within this sector it should be considered that an understanding of inter-personal relations and psychological processes involving boundaries and inter-relatedness should become a high priority.

Cultural Issues

Cultural issues are identified in the management of these patients which goes beyond the racial and ethnic issues usually covered in the literature and embraces cultures for example in relation to drug abusers. Often health sector staff spoke of patients been transferred from the criminal justice system with "a prison culture and attitude". This often referred to individuals who continued to refer to nursing staff as "screws", were anti-authoritarian, often non-compliant to treatment and antagonistic to staff.

Nursing staff often struggled to understand the complexities of difficult groups such as young, inner city, streetwise drug abusers as well as the more complex issues surrounding racial and ethnic differences. The management of substance abuse within the system concerns both sectors and is a growing problem for staff responding to patients behaving in a disturbed and bizarre manner. The traditional response to these episodes has often been rapid tranquillisation combined with restraint and /or seclusion. Staff need to be vigilant to the possibility that patient presenting in a bizarre or difficult manner might be accessing illicit substances rather than suffering from a psychotic or psychological disturbance, and interventions and management of situations should reflect that. Of particular concern from the study was an apparent poor level and understanding of intervention techniques such as de-escalation in the prison system, and the lack of consistency in practice with interventions in the health sector.

Complaints

Many staff raised concerns about and criticised, the current systems in both sectors of the management of complaints by patients. It should be noted that the number of complaints received from difficult patients is high compared with the overall patient population. In its evidence to the Fallon Inquiry (Ashworth Hospital 1997) the hospital cited that "At Ashworth. Male PD patients represent, on average, 28% of the male population and they were responsible for making 43% of the complaints received during the period October 1996 to September 1997".

The issues of frivolous and malicious complaints is prevalent across the world. It is a major problem in the United States because of the emphasis placed upon the protection of the rights of the individual under the Constitution.

Every patient has the right to complain and to pursue his or her complaint through the formal procedure. This is strongly reinforced in our findings through various processes in both the health and criminal justice system. Many issues pursued through the procedure would not necessarily be highlighted if patients chose not to complain or felt they were unable to complain. It is concerning, however, that despite significant progress in dealing with complaints, staff are often faced with an inflexible process which emphasises procedure, rather than the individual patient and his/her clinical need. In the case of persistent and mischievous complainants this can only serve to raise expectations beyond what is reasonable, in many cases it can be counter therapeutic and overall places a considerable strain on resources.

The NHS Trust Federation 'Working Hard to Please' identified the problem of persistent/vexatious complainants in a recent evaluation of the NHS Complaints Procedure which stated that there appeared to be no brake in vexatious complainants. The potential for more malicious complaints is heightened in a secure environment, therefore much effort is given to reassuring patients and staff of the rigours of the complaints investigation process. Working in an environment where patients are more likely to conspire against staff or to coerce or manipulate other patients in an effort to 'get at' staff can cause considerable strain.

There is evidence that such complaints are made against staff who are appropriately carrying out procedures or taking decisions based on the clinical needs of the patient. This understandably causes a great deal of anxiety and frustration to staff working in these conditions on a daily basis. Additionally, there are patients who make no effort to pursue complaints at ward or departmental level, believing satisfaction will only be achieved by pursuing complaints at the highest level.

Although a relatively small number of patients reflect these concerns, they are a significant minority who make tremendous demands on the service and serve only to devalue the complaint process. As one in three complaints are about nursing care in the health sector, nursing managers spend a vast amount of time either interviewing staff or supporting staff through the complaints process.

<u>Additional Comments</u>

Without doubt the complexities of behaviour and difficulties presented by this significant minority require a high level of teamwork and consistency of approach in the day-to-day management of their care. The nursing staff sometimes feel that they take the brunt of dysfunctional or disorganised clinical teams. These often highly confrontational patients can make it difficult for staff to ensure a safe environment is maintained as they will often repeatedly challenge security procedures, particularly room and body searches, as an infringement of their rights, particularly within the health sector. It has been a useful development for secure environments that the issue of searching has been recently clarified in the Court following a challenge by patients from Broadmoor Hospital. Guidance has now been issued from the Mental Health Act Commission by way of the revised Code of Practice.

Concern was also expressed, both in the health and prison sectors, about the use of agency and bank nurses in secure environments. There was a strong belief that this undermined consistency and they presented as a potentially vulnerable group which could be exploited by difficult patients: however no empirical evidence to support this assertion. The final key theme related to the staff themselves and the consistent problem of the was low level of support available to staff in dealing with difficult patients either from a line management perspective or in the availability of clinical supervision.

Staff with long-standing experience of working in these environments felt generally undervalued and the skills they had developed were poorly recognised. They believed that there was an over-reliance by managers on academic qualifications. It was clear that some experienced staff have experientially developed methods of working successfully in this complex environment and could be a source of great help to new members of staff and in the development of further training, they present in some instances an untapped resource.

There are no immediate solutions for the management of this difficult group of patients. Their negative impact can be minimised however by training staff appropriately, the provision of appropriate physical and human environments with attention to such issues as grade and skill mix, effective support and supervision systems within a framework of robust evidence based policies and procedures which are protective for both staff and patients.

Conclusions

The focus groups and focus interviews provided much of the evidence regarding the difficulties faced by practitioners when working with specific client groups. The main client groups which emerged as presenting particular challenges were those clients with personality disorder, substance abuse, women's issues and self-harm. The following issues were identified:

- The nursing of patients with personality disorders transcends both prison and secure mental health care and presents major challenges for nurses in both settings.

- In effect, nurses in secure services are charged with providing care for a large group of individuals with particularly challenging behaviours but whose disorders are ill defined, whose treatment is often haphazard and the outcomes for whom, in relation to clinical targets, are poorly understood and progress difficult to measure.

- The therapeutic goal set for many patients in these settings is about improving the management of patients rather than necessarily improving the clinical condition itself. This is highly relevant to a consideration of the goals of nursing interventions.

- The issue of the 'relationship' when caring for personality disorder is poorly understood as its effect in compromising professional boundaries.

- Particular clarity is needed to understand the dynamics of confidentiality and autonomy when nursing patients with personality disorders.

- Mental health care is based on the establishment of a therapeutic relationship. Institutional life, particularly in the long term settings of many forensic services, may mean that nursing staff are placed in situations that test boundaries or provide a degree of informality that may threaten the necessary therapeutic endeavour.

- There should be greater proliferation, training and support of risk management strategies in relation to self-harm. This should include a greater awareness of environmental factors and diagnostic issues.

- Greater emphasis should be given to developing evidence-based practice for decision making following self-harm incidents.

- There should be a requirement for all nursing staff working in secure environments to receive clinical support and supervision on a regular basis.

- Nursing staff should be supported by a robust system of operational policies and procedures, which are known to all, subject to regular monitoring and update, and supported and reinforced by management.

- There is a need for an appropriate level of environmental and human resource provision with attention to such issues as grade and skill mix, effective support and supervision systems within a framework of robust evidence based policies and procedures which are protective for both patients and staff.

- Although a relatively small number of patients are persistent /vexatious complainants, they are a significant minority who make tremendous demands on the service and serve only to devalue the complaint process.

- The challenge for nurses is to provide a care and treatment service for patients but this is difficult when energy and resources are channelled into operating defensively. Responses to issues tend to involve uncoordinated action rather than focused, considered thought and debate.

4.6 Identify the extent to which existing Council policies are utilised and inform practice within secure environments

The ethical dilemmas presented in practice settings

A profession is defined not only by its body of expertise, but also its values and ethics (Dale *et al.* 1999). Medical ethics codes are among the oldest recorded professional codes. Consistent throughout them are the principles that the health of the patient will be the first consideration, that human dignity will always be respected, and concepts of dedication to the service of humanity generally. Such codes and concepts include care of the profession and fellow professionals, in the senses of being honest and committed to furthering knowledge and its application in the field. The corollary is that intentional harm to those seeking help from physicians, lack of respect for them as people, or action in unnecessary ignorance are all unacceptable, and breaches of professional codes. Within health services, trained personnel other than doctors have generally now adopted similar codes and formed professions too. Within the criminal justice system, lawyers have long had such professional standing, but other disciplines, for example the probation service, are now also joining these ranks.

Working within secure clinical environments presents healthcare professionals with a challenging and diverse role that embraces a range of issues demanding ethical consideration.

Secure mental health services are subjected to a great deal of public attention. Much of the (frequently negative) exposure that they receive relates to either the nature of the patient group, the facilities in which they are detained or the perceived attitudes of those who choose to work in such a specialism (Chaloner 1998).

The recent emergence of healthcare ethics as an academic discipline has reflected the growing interest in the moral aspects of all forms of healthcare delivery.

It might be thought that an understanding of ethics could resolve the moral dilemmas encountered in practice. However, an awareness of ethics can only guide effective practice and assist in finding informed responses to ethical decisions.

Singer points out "... ethics is not an ideal system that is noble in theory but no good in practice. The reverse of this is closer to the truth ... for the whole point of ethical judgements is to guide practice". (Singer 1993).

Ethics provides a framework for examining the morality of human behaviour beyond a somewhat simplistic distinction between 'right' and 'wrong', ethics as applied to practice demands an understanding of important ethical concepts (e.g. confidentiality), ethically important decision-making procedures (e.g. deciding when confidentiality should be maintained), the ability to apply such concepts and decision-making procedures to real-life cases plus effective communication abilities (Gillon 1996).

Issues have been raised about the social control aspect of secure mental health institutions, 'The shortening of the periods of detention for treatment, deterrence or retribution have made a live issue of whether (or when) it is justifiable to detain violent and sexual offenders solely for the protection of others' (Walker 1991). Issues of social control are especially pertinent to the management of offender patients beyond the secure mental health setting (Mason and Mercer 1996).

While it is obviously the case that an individual's physical movements are restricted in a secure environment this does not necessarily imply that they lack autonomy or lose the capacity to think, decide and act on the basis of such thought and decision freely and independently' (Gillon 1985). Bodies such as the Mental Health Act Commission protect the legal rights of patients, but their 'moral' rights, e.g. the right to the truth, seem less clear.

The majority of effective healthcare interventions are dependent on the informed consent of patients. (McLean 1989) The imbalance in the carer/patient relationship suggests that the active participation in therapeutic programmes may be reliant on a degree of coercion, even if this is not intended. Patients may be motivated to co-operate with treatment and therapeutic programmes for pragmatic reasons in relation to the prospect of earlier discharge or transfer from hospital. (Chaloner 1998)

For some nurses a relatively small number of patients may not appear to accord with an accepted view of mental disorder. For example, Personality Disorders may not readily fulfil commonly applied and culturally accepted criteria for 'illness' or 'disease' and it may be claimed that there is an inherent difficulty in attempting to attribute directly either term to the personality disordered patients' condition.

An assessment of whether such individuals are indeed 'mad or bad' (Bavidge 1989) and whether such terms accurately reflect the nature of their disorder may determine what managerial approach should be adopted - health care or imprisonment/ punishment.

The most frequently considered ethical issues are those that impact directly on daily practice. The somewhat sparse literature pertaining to the ethics of forensic mental health nursing tends to focus on such practical concerns.

Chaloner (1998) outlines five areas of practical moral issues that nurses face in working in secure environments. These include: power and control, for example, the use of restraint including seclusion (Lehane and Rees 1996, Alty 1997); risk assessment and the prediction of dangerousness (Allen 1997), consent to treatment (Clarke 1998), confidentiality, and 'Unpopular' patients.

Chaloner (1998) suggests that "An adherence to professional codes and guidelines (UKCC 1992b, 1996), can assist in finding a solution to moral dilemmas. However, a strict adherence to such codes, while professionally appropriate, does not provide an adequate replacement for a fully considered ethical appraisal of a particular situation."

UKCC Standards and Guidelines

A recent report commissioned by the UKCC (Gilmore 1998) identifies that there is very little robust evaluative literature relating to the usage and effectiveness of UKCC standards and guidelines by practitioners (Redfem 1997, Tadd 1997). The findings from the Gilmore study provide a background for the scoping exercise, particularly these issues in secure environments.

The limited evidence available indicates that the complexities identified in disseminating and implementing clinical guidelines are likely to apply to all UKCC standards and guidelines. The study by Jowett *et al.* (1997) has already identified problems with dissemination and implementation of the Scope of Professional Practice.

What evidence exists regarding the efficacy of UKCC standards and guidelines tends to be conflicting (Gilmore 1998). "This problem is compounded by ineffective dissemination and implementation strategies ... the research question could be: are we providing effective standards and guidelines to registrants and are they (and the patients) appearing to benefit from them?"

Preliminary evidence, from a telephone survey (Gilmore 1998) indicated that NHS nurse directors saw it as their responsibility to implement some UKCC standards and guidelines locally. These standards inform the formation of local policies relating to nursing/midwifery/health visiting staff. Examples of these are nursing strategies, guidelines for records and record keeping, standards for the administration of medicines and standards for professional practice and conduct. UKCC standards/guidelines tend to be monitored indirectly through local audits of these policies. In general, employees are expected to know practice in accordance with the UKCC code of conduct. Specific strategies mentioned for monitoring practitioners practice and conduct were Individual Performance Review (IPR), critical incidents (such as drug errors, customer complaints) and clinical supervision (suggested by one respondent).

The level and type of responsibilities of respondents is thought to influence the extent of knowledge and type of usage of UKCC standards and guidelines (nursing/midwifery senior managers versus practitioners whose main role is direct patient care).

There is a paucity of evidence evaluating the impact of UKCC standards and guidelines on practitioners or their practice. Selective literature reviews by Redfem (1997) and Tadd (1997) identified very little empirical investigations of practitioner knowledge and usage of The Scope of Professional Practice (UKCC 1992) and the Code of Professional Conduct (UKCC 1992) respectively.

A study of nurses' and midwives' knowledge of the Code of Professional Conduct (UKCC 1992) by Whyte and Gajos (1996) found a lack of clarity about how, to whom and for what they are accountable. There was little evidence that the Code informed their decision-making. These findings are corroborated by evidence from a qualitative study by Lipp (1998). Lipp (1998) aimed to identify ethical decision making methods used by nurses in clinical areas and reported that participants made no mention of the UKCC guidelines as an everyday support for ethical decision making. The authors suggests that this could be explained by the intuitive approach adapted by the informants whereby they know something influenced the decision but are unable to articulate the precise source of support. Certain factors such as doctors, colleagues and the organisation, were reported to profoundly influence ethical decision-making.

Most of the literature identified, which addresses benefits to patients of UKCC standards and guidelines, focuses on the Scope of Professional Practice (UKCC 1992b). Rose *et al.* (1997) conducted a literature review to assess the extended role of the nurse especially in ophthalmology. The general theme to emerge is that one cannot assume that nurses who extend their role are competent to do so. The research raised concerns about the safety of role extension in ophthalmic settings and the implications are that there must also be questions about the safety of nurses expanding their practice in other areas without specialist qualifications. Newbold (1996) has also raised the dangers in unregulated nursing roles.

The literature searches yielded very few papers or articles, which deal with either the dissemination of UKCC standards and guidelines, or how they are implemented locally. Most of the evidence available on the effectiveness of methods of dissemination and implementation of clinical guidelines relates to medicine (Cheater and Closs 1997).

Examination of the medical literature shows that dissemination of guidelines alone is usually insufficient to change clinical behaviour (Grimshaw and Russell 1993b, Grimshaw *et al.* 1995). The following table shows the rate of probability of guidelines being successfully utilised. The chances of implementation are significantly increased if guidelines have been developed within the organisation and the implementation strategy includes education of the participants involved and is patient specific. Chances of success are reduced when people, or organisations, not in direct contact with those whom the guidelines affect undertake the development of guidelines.

Dissemination and implementation strategies also have an impact on success levels. Postal information to recipients of guidelines is far less successful than face to face contact. Including guidelines in educational packages has proved to increase the levels of uptake of guidelines.

Relative probability of being effective	Development strategy	Dissemination strategy	Implementation Strategy
High	Internal	Specific educational intervention	Patient specific reminder at time of consultation
Above average	Intermediate	Continuing education	Patient specific feedback
Below average	External local	Posting targeted groups	General feedback
Low	External national	Publication in professional journal	General reminder of guideline

Table 4.6.1 Factors influencing the successful introduction of guidelines
(Cited in Grimshaw and Russell 1994)

In order to provide up-to-date information and monitor trends, a 300-person telephone survey was undertaken by the UKCC in early 1999. This represented a balanced survey in that the 300 people were representative of the register in terms of country, gender and parts of the register. In fact, in order to test the views of mental health nurses and midwives in particular, there was over-representation of them in the survey

On the two new publications that were the subject of the survey, Guidelines on Records and Record Keeping and Guidelines for Mental Health and Learning Disability, responses were positive. Some 83% said they had received the guidelines on record keeping and, of these,

90% found them useful (98% for midwives). On the mental health guidelines, 61% had read them and, of these, 95% found them useful.

On the role of the UKCC, people saw the organisation as a standard-setting body, a regulatory body, and a governing body. There was no real identification of areas of work that the UKCC should be doing but isn't now.

Findings

During the Scoping exercise the findings from the previous UKCC studies have been used to identify comparisons and differences of views amongst nurses in secure environments. The instruments used by the UKCC to gather data in 1997 and 1999 were incorporated into the organisational and staff questionnaires, and were also used within the audit process.

Some participants in the focus groups identified a potential need for some of the UKCC publications to be contextualised for working in secure settings, these included the code of conduct and administration of medications. A significant number of nurses working in prison expressed the view that the UKCC should acknowledge this area of practice on the Notification of Practice forms when a nurse renews their registration.

The staff questionnaires from the Prison Services and secure hospital provision revealed that Guidelines for records and record keeping had been read by 72% of nurses working in prison and 83.6% hospital nurses with 61.3% and 71.6% respectively finding it useful. For the Mental Health Guidelines only 36.3% of nurses working in prison and 57.1% of hospital nurses having read it and 31.1% and 50.2% respectively finding it useful. One reason this low response is possibly because the Mental Health and Learning Disabilities Guidelines were not distributed to general nurses who make up a high proportion of Nurses working in prison.

Staff Responses

Figure 4.6.1 UKCC Publications- Read

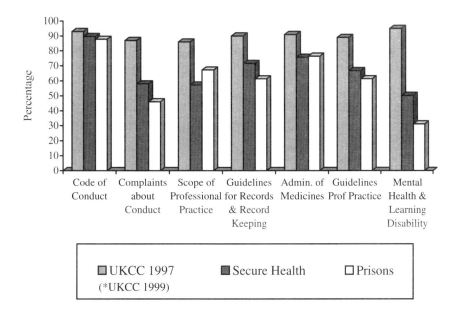

127

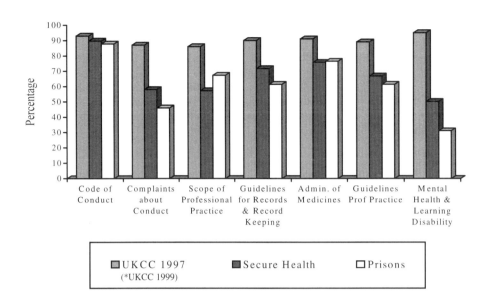

Figure 4.6.2 UKCC Publications- Found Useful

The graphs represent responses from 714 individual nurses as to whether the UKCC publications had been read (Figure 4.6.1) and whether the nurse had found them useful (Figure 4.6.2). The data has been compared with surveys undertaken by the UKCC in 1997 and 1999.

The general consensus from nurses involved in the scoping exercise is that UKCC policies and guidelines provide a systematic framework for their professional practice. The majority of contributors and respondents were aware of current documents and indicated that policies and protocols within their employing organisations tended to adhere to the principles within the guidelines. In the main the UKCC publications were available in the workplace, but a number of organisations had not replaced the Standards for Records and Record Keeping with the Guidelines document. The low response to the Guidelines for Mental Health and Learning Disabilities nursing is because RGNs working in the Prison Services would not have received this document as it was only automatically circulated to nurses on the UKCC register with a mental health or learning disability qualification.

During the focus groups many of the participants expressed a view that the standards and guidelines were not easily applied in a secure setting because of the nature of the client group or because of the culture of the organisation.

Results from the Organisational Questionnaire

Representatives of organisations were asked which UKCC policies and procedure were utilised within their organisation. The responses indicated that an extremely high proportion of the 115 organisations that responded had received and utilised UKCC standards and guidelines, but during the audits many of the sites visited did not have current copies of UKCC publications available in the ward areas or health centres. For example 11 of the 18 sites did not have copies of the Guidelines for Records and Record Keeping, although some did have copies of Standards for Records and Record keeping which the Guidelines replaced. 11 sites did not have direct access to Guidelines regarding confidentiality, 5 sites could not produce copies of the Standards for the Administration of Medications. Although 16 sites did have copies of the Code of Professional Conduct, failed to produce copies of the Scope of Professional Practice, and only 11 had copies of PREP guidelines.

Application of UKCC Standards and Guidelines within the Prison Services

The main area where there is real or potential conflict is in some areas of the prison sector where it is not always possible for nurses to completely meet UKCC standards. Although the UKCC Code of Professional Conduct is referenced in the England and Wales Standing Order 13 (Healthcare) in paragraph 8 which is appropriate to the majority of nurses working in prisons it states that: "The Health Care Manager (the most senior nursing officer by grade) is responsible to the managing medical officer for the performance of the nursing services and the maintenance of standards of nursing care which accord with the Code of Professional Conduct of the United Kingdom Central Council for Nursing, Midwifery and Health Visiting. He or she is responsible, in consultation with the Managing Medical Officer, to the Governor for the general conduct of the nursing staff". In Scotland nurses are managed by nurses.

The most frequently quoted examples were in relation to access to prisoners and the administration of medications. Because of the regimes in place within the prison there are occasions when a nurse has to administer medications on the prison wing whilst a prisoner is in his/her cell. This means that the nurse cannot ensure that the medication has been taken or whether it has been secreted.

Walsh (1998) cites Wilmott (1997), who suggests that one of the main challenges to the nurse in prison is caring for inmates to whom access is denied. Although nurses may carry prison keys to allow freedom of movement around the prison, there are times during the day when in the interests of security, access to inmates is curtailed or denied. Most prisons lock all inmates in their cells at certain times during the day and all night. Wilmott reported that security staff may be reluctant to use their powers to open a cell at the nurses' request. Similarly, McMillan (1997) reported an extreme example where in one prison at night the nurse did not have cell keys. A prison officer and a prison officer with a prison dog were called before access to a cell was given to the nurse, although this is not common practice in the majority of prisons it is cited as an example of the problems occasionally faced by nurses when they need to provide nursing care.

The positive identification of prisoners, in some institutions, where there is a high turnover of inmates, causes concerns. The problem has been solved in many prisons where on reception the prisoner is issued with either an identity card or other form of positive identification, which can be used when nurses are administering medications.

Another area that causes conflict is in relation to "in-possession " medication. A number of nurses cited examples of prisoners being given "in-possession " medication when attending court or other external visits only to have discipline officers removing the medication from the prisoner in order to "minimise risk".

At the 1997 RCN Annual Congress, a motion was passed requesting that the UKCC to develop a Code of Practice specifically for nurses working in prison. The motion was overwhelmingly supported with 446 votes for and 38 against. A spokesperson for the RCN mental health society, felt that the difficulties faced by nurses working in prison in adhering to the Code of Conduct were a fault of the prison service and not the Code of Conduct, (Nursing Times editorial 1997). He mentioned that some nurses are not familiar with the breadth of nurse's accountability and therefore are unable to exercise this accountability in informing their employers about their difficulties. Lyne (1997) in her discussion of prison health care mentioned the general perception of prison Governors "remaining to be convinced of a clear way forward for staffing health care centres and nurses having to work in conditions which fail to meet their UKCC Code of Professional Conduct. (Walsh 1998)

Walsh (1998) examined in detail the Code of Professional Conduct and suggests that some of the clauses within it appear on face value to be quite incompatible with the care of patients and development of nursing practice within the prison environment. She explored some of these clauses and compared them to the literature concerning prison nursing.

"Clause 1 of the Code of Professional Conduct states: *"Act always in such a manner as to promote and safeguard the interests and well being of patients and clients."*

Whilst clause 2 states: *"Ensure that no action or omission on your part or within your sphere of responsibility, is detrimental to the interests, condition or safety of patients and clients"*.

In England and Wales, nurses working in prison, as part of the prison staff have a duty to maintain order, control and discipline. Prison rule 47 specifies areas of misconduct and breaches of discipline under which inmates can be charged. A consequence of violating rule 47 is an adjudication or hearing in front of the prison Governor which, if the inmate is found guilty, often leads to a punishment. Nurses as employees can instigate an adjudication at which they are then called to give evidence. Prisoners even if located in the prison hospital are subject to prison rules and the consequences for violating those rules. This leads to a situation in which nurses may become involved in the punishment of their patients.

Some nurses in the prison service in England and Wales, are also involved in assisting the prison doctor in deciding if a prisoner is fit to attend an adjudication and hence fit for the punishment, which may result. Dulfer (1992) makes reference to these duties which nurses working in prison perform and states that nurses do not find it easy. Alternatively, the nurse could well be safeguarding the interests of the inmate in that they could protect an unfit inmate from punishment.

As was mentioned earlier, prisons have certain times of the day and all night when all inmates must be locked in their cells. This is adhered to without exception as security necessitates it. However, in some prisons, difficulties may arise for the nurse in that the depressed, suicidal or distressed patient must also be locked up. Access to the patient is a problem in adhering to clauses 1 and 2 as locking a suicidal patient in an unfurnished room is debatable as to its usefulness for the patient. Depressed, anxious and upset patients may not benefit psychologically from being locked in a prison cell. However, these actions are necessary in a prison during these patrol states and it is often the nurse who must lock the patient in the cell. In some prisons, throughout the United Kingdom, this issue has been addressed, but it remains a key issue for many nurses.

Clause 10 of the Code of Professional Conduct is concerned with the management of confidential information.

In the prison setting, the nurse must make a number of decisions regarding information given to him/her in the course of their duties. It must be remembered that it is not only purely medical information that is given to the nurse. Nurses in prison carry out non-clinical duties and often receive information from inmates. A decision must be made by the nurse as to whether a duty of confidentiality is inferred and/or assumed by the prisoner simply because of the nurses role and a subsequent duty of confidentiality to patients.

Nurses may be called upon to care for inmates who have been attacked or even raped by others (Day 1983). Questions arise here for the nurse as the inmate may discuss the attack with the nurse. The nurse must decide whether to share the information with other staff or not, possibly putting the victim in further danger but consequently perhaps protecting other inmates.

Another facet to confidentiality in prison concerns the sharing of information with other staff in the prison. Prison Officers, chaplains, psychologists, doctors, probation officers and even the citizens advice bureau all have a role to play in the overall care of the inmate whilst in prison. Prison officers interact with inmates 24 hours a day and could be described as "significant others" in the context of Orem's (1985) self-care model of nursing. The nurse must decide whether information gained from the inmate, medical or otherwise is to be part of the officer's knowledge of the prisoner.

Confidentiality may be breached in the interests of the inmate in some instances where an inmate's location within the prison is influenced by the inmate's medical condition. For example, inmates with epilepsy are placed in shared accommodation for their own safety. Their cellmate may also be informed of the inmates' condition and taught about what to do if the inmate has a fit. This is vital as the inmate may fit during a patrol state in which case the actions of the cellmate may be crucial to the safety of the inmate. Some medical conditions must also be disclosed to the labour board, when an inmate is seeking employment and also to the kitchen staff who may need to prepare special meals such as diabetic meals.

From the work undertaken, the main problems associated in complying with, and application of UKCC standards and guidelines appear to be for some nurses working in the Prison Services. These nurses concerns emerge as the result of some nurses, in England Wales and Northern Ireland, undertaking a dual role - that of both carer and custodian. Although the recent report from the Prison Services and NHS Executive recommends that the custodial role is separated from the nursing role, the nurse cannot remove the need for security from their role both in physical and relational security.

The Standards for the Administration of Medications (UKCC 1992), together with the *Review of Prescribing, Supply and Administration of Medicines* (The Crown Report, Department of Health 1999), provides a framework for safe administration of medications to prisoners. Although some action has been taken to develop appropriate pharmaceutical services the Prison Services need to develop protocols and practices which are applied consistently and meet the needs of prisoners and the prisons. Doing this will minimise the conflict that some nurses face in trying to work to UKCC standards.

Conclusions

Questionnaires, audits and focus groups provided useful information about the extent to which UKCC policies were available, utilised and assisted in the development of practice within secure settings. The following issues were identified :

- UKCC registrants need to be more readily appraised of existing UKCC guidelines.

- The UKCC should work with employers in these settings to ensure that practitioners understand and apply the principles already developed and contribute to the development of new guidelines.

- Without UKCC policies and values being more fully accessed and integrated the dominant resource for ethical decision making will continue to be organisational and cultural norms.

- The evidence suggests that the penetration of UKCC documents is incomplete. The relative usefulness and applicability of some documents is questioned. *(Code of Professional Conduct, Standards for Administration of Medicines)*

- The ability of nurses to maintain professional standards in the safe administration of medicines is particularly complicated by security considerations and regimes within the Prison Services.

- There is a perception that standards and guidelines set by the UKCC may not adequately address the needs of nurses working with patients presenting at behavioural extremes or who challenge professional boundaries.

- Nurses require additional support in ethical decision making when applying security measures and in instigating investigation or disciplinary actions against prisoners.

- Organisational requirements within the Prison Services appear to constrain the ability of nurses to utilise some UKCC policies to inform practice. An example of which would be issues around medication management and health assessment in the prison services.

4.7 Identify practice issues relevant to the physical health needs of these populations; care of women (including care of pregnant women); care of people from different cultural backgrounds

The rate of physical illness among individuals with diagnosed psychiatric conditions has been found to be higher than that in the general population. Kratzer Worley *et al.* (1990) found that psychiatric inpatients had significantly higher incidence and prevalence rates for physical illnesses than psychiatric outpatients did. While these data may be attributed partially to more thorough medical examinations in inpatient units, they give support for the more thorough assessment of physical health status among severely mentally ill persons. Their use of general health care services is limited.

Psychiatric patients who seek help for medically related symptoms are sometimes seen as disruptive and often illnesses can go undiagnosed for a variety of reasons. Problems that do not fall into the defined category for treatment, i.e. mental illness, often fail to be recognised and addressed as mental health practitioners are not always thoroughly trained or encouraged to identify additional physical health needs or problems. (Hall *et al.* 1982)

Holmberg (1988) identified a number of specific physical illnesses that were associated with long term mental illness and/or institutional care, these included: cardiovascular and endocrine disorders, medication side-effects (obesity and tardive dyskinesia). Some patients were also found to have co-existing somatic disorders such as seizures, coronary and respiratory disease and diabetes. In general, these problems were usually mis/undiagnosed with outpatients or those in secure environments for short periods of time, the longer people are in patients the more likely physical changes were diagnosed and treated.

Accessing health care can be problematic, even if the individual is not actively psychotic, the negative symptoms of chronic mental illness such as passivity, withdrawal and depression may inhibit motivation to seek care.

In 1997 the Office for National Statistics carried out a survey to look at the Psychiatric morbidity amongst prisoners in England and Wales that included an analysis of the physical health needs of this population. The findings indicated that about a third of male prisoners and two fifths of female prisoners reported a long-standing physical complaint. Among men, musculo-skeletal complaints were the most common followed by respiratory complaints, whereas among women this order was reversed. The only variables significantly associated with having a physical complaint were age (the likelihood of having a physical complaint increased with age), sex (Women were more likely than men to report a physical complaint) and the presence of significant neurotic symptoms or evidence of functional psychosis.

The importance of attending to the physical health needs of these clients has been affirmed within the Scottish Prison Service Standards for the Health Care of Prisoners (SPS 1998) where assessment, evaluation and triage are key factors, and the American Nurses Association (1982) in its Standards of Psychiatric Nursing Practice.

Respondents with significant neurotic symptoms were more likely than other prisoners to report a physical complaint. However, those with evidence of psychosis were less likely to report physical health problems compared with prisoners without a psychotic disorder.

Research has shown high levels of mental disorder and drug misuse and general poor health among prisoners (Gunn *et al.* 1991). Drug dependence in the year before coming into prison particularly dependence on opiates, was associated with increased reporting of an infectious disease compared with those who were not drug-dependent.

Women in prison

Women are a small proportion of the total population of prisoners. As a result, their interests and needs are often overlooked by a service which is geared more towards dealing with male prisoners. (Squires & Stobl 1996). In 1992, women were convicted for 40,000 indictable offences and the female prison population stood at 1,577. In 1996 this figure fell to 38,000 and there were 2,262 women in prison. By March 13th 1998, there were 3,068 women in prison which has now increased to approximately 3,200 (Feb 1999)-the highest female prison population this century.

"The majority of incarcerated women come from impoverished backgrounds ... are addicted to drugs or alcohol, have not been exposed to or been able to access health care on a regular basis, have emotional and mental health problems, or have significant histories of physical and sexual abuse"(Maeve 1997). As a result their health needs include basic health care, teaching, counselling and supportive care (Wilson and Leasure 1991) and the most frequent problems include: drug/alcohol addiction, gynaecological disease and exacerbation of chronic health problems, particularly hypertension, diabetes and epilepsy. (Wilson and Leasure 1991, Osborne 1995)

Pregnant Women in Prison

The care of pregnant women in prison is an issue which causes much emotion, both within the services and in the media, equally for the well being of the women concerned, and the babies to be born to these women whilst they are serving a prison sentence.

Since 1948, imprisoned women have delivered their babies outside the prisons - unless delivery happens too quickly. The service for pregnant women is based on the United Nations' Standard Minimum Rules for the Treatment of Prisoners.

There are a number of groups who are opposed to pregnant women, or even women with young dependant children, being imprisoned under any circumstances. "Many present day reformers consider the imprisoning of mothers with small children to be a barbaric practice: the Royal College of Midwives has joined the Howard League in stating publicly that no pregnant women or mother of a small child should be behind bars, with or without her baby." (Devlin 1998) However, given that this is unlikely to be achieved in the short term the important issue for many is the improved care of this often-ignored population.

There are, at present, four mother and baby units in prisons in England, with places for around 68 babies. In two of these Units babies can remain with their mothers until they are nine months old, and in the other two until they are eighteen months old. Cornton Vale, in Scotland, has developed a protocol, which has established mother and baby rooms at Peebles House.

The public debate concerning pregnant women was fuelled by the case of Susan Edwards, of whom it was reported that she was handcuffed whilst giving birth in 1994. The then Home Secretary apologised for this and stated that this situation would never occur again. Then, in 1995, the Prison Services Security Manual introduced the guidelines for the routine handcuffing of women prisoners under escort. The following quote deals specifically with pregnant prisoners. " If handcuffs are removed it must be only at the request of a doctor or midwife attending a birth and it must be done only for the shortest time; that is from immediately before the treatment or examination begins, or when labour begins" (Ogden 1995). This indicates that women will always be handcuffed in the first instance, and the restraints be removed only at the insistence of a medical professional. Women in Prison (1999) express a view that the use of physical restraints such as handcuffs and chains contravenes the United Nations guidance that 'chains shall not be used as a method of restraint',

" It seems we are going to have to wait until the European Convention of Human Rights is incorporated into British Law before a challenge can be raised" (Women in Prison 1999).

It is well documented that the majority of women in prison are from deprived backgrounds, which often results in poor general health, and an increased risk of complications during pregnancy. Osborne (1995), Maeve (1997), and Scott and Blantern (1998) validate these concerns and Wilson and Leasure (1991) outline exactly what these deprivations can result in. Pregnant women in prison "are at risk from pregnancy complications and poor outcomes of pregnancy. Often, the women have an obstetric history of complications and are in poor general health, nutritionally compromised and economically deprived. Their lifestyle has frequently included alcohol and drug abuse, inadequate health care and exposure to numerous infectious diseases, increasing the risk of poor pregnancy outcomes." (Wilson and Leasure 1991)

Pregnant women are kept in the main wings of the prison. (In Holloway they have the choice to be moved to a special unit, but most choose not to.) They have regular access to ante-natal classes and specialist health care professionals: however, different prisons report variable frequency of these services. (Howard League for Prison Reform 1995)

In the past, the care of a pregnant prisoner whilst under escort was left to the discretion of security, rather than medical staff. This resulted in situations where women were restrained with closeting chains whilst in windowless toilets, with the staff waiting outside. However, due in part to the actions of pressure groups and the media, this situation is improving. In women's prisons today the midwife ensures that all interviews and examinations are undertaken in privacy, which means prison officers wait outside, and that prisoners are escorted by female officers whilst on visits. (Scott and Blantern 1998) However, it is to be noted that this was dependent on sufficient staff being available and subject to the patient not being deemed a security risk. In this instance then, restraints will still be used and prison officers may remain present during all stages of the pregnancy and birth process, each case being decided on its own merit.

Action is being taken to address this issue, a report from the England and Wales Prison Service (HM Prison Service 1999) identifies the need to review the restrictions placed on eligibility for places in Mother and Baby Units, to provide crèche facilities so that mothers can work or study. They also state that the best interests of the baby should be at the heart of the Prison Service's procedures for Mother and Baby Units.

In Prisons across the UK work has already been undertaken to make positive changes in the way mothers and babies are catered for within the Prison Services. Styal Prison has developed protocols in collaboration with the midwifery services of their local NHS Trust. The aim of the service is to "provide midwifery care which is woman-centred, recognises and is sensitive to the needs of each individual woman with the emphasis on choice, continuity and control throughout the pregnancy continuum, at the same time ensuring accessibility of all services." (Kitzinger 1999)

Cornton Vale, in Scotland, has an established Maternity Care Provision that includes access to a named Midwife, the appointment of a Health Visitor and links with the Social Work Department.

Holloway has introduced the 'Holloway Doula Group'. ('Doula' is a Greek word for a woman who helps another in childbirth). Sheila Kitzinger became aware of the needs of women prisoners who were having babies and took action with others to end the use of handcuffs in childbirth. The plight of prisoners giving birth without any support from friends and family also became clear. Sheila's article in the National Childbirth Trust Teachers' Mailing inspired a voluntary group of London-based ante-natal teachers to set up the 'Holloway Doula Group'. A prisoner's mother says:

"When I arrived at the hospital I was surprised to see a woman comforting and cherishing my daughter. She not only stayed for the birth but she and another 'birth sister' helped with the care of mother and baby throughout their time in hospital. They are the most selfless people I have ever met."

Women are made aware of the Doula system through ante-natal classes, literature distributed and displayed in the prison and other involved groups. Any woman who requests support is sent guidelines and is visited by a member of the Holloway Doula Group who gets to know her and discusses with her a birth plan. When she goes into labour, she is met at the hospital and stays with her continuously through labour. If necessary, other members of the group also support her during the birth and in the days she spends in hospital. The Doula Group aim to do this for every woman from Holloway prison who requests their services.

A prisoner writes:

"I was made to feel at ease and even though in a lot of pain I was conscious of her always being there. I had more faith and trust in my birthing partner than anyone else .... You guys have rebuilt my trust and faith in human nature."

Women in Secure Hospitals

Women in secure hospitals share a common problem with women in the Prison sector. Travers and Aiyegbusi (1998) report that childhood neglect and trauma overlap with self neglect and self harm in later life. Both self neglect and self harm by patients can be seen as antecedents to significant physical health problems. Complications associated with eating disorders have led to this population experiencing problems ranging from extremes of anaemia and malnutrition to morbid obesity.

Chain smoking, which is quite commonplace, undoubtedly exacerbates respiratory problems such as asthma which is present in a high percentage of patients. Women patients present with an increased level of endocrine pathology in the form of thyroid, diabetic and reproductive system disorders. Travers and Aiyegbusi (1998) support the view of van der Kolk and McFarlane (1996) who suggest there is a relationship between a restricted ability to express emotions verbally and impaired immune system functioning which in turn relates to physical illness. They also noted that the women patients tend to suffer many infections which lead to antibiotic treatments.

Ethnic minorities

Across the UK, the specific needs of ethnic minority patients are frequently overlooked when resources are allocated. Their needs are not always addressed during the education of health-care professionals and they lose out when health-care services are delivered. (Watson 1990)

The responses from the organisational questionnaires show a variance between the prison service and the health care sector in relation to the development and implementation of policies for minority groups.

Table 4.7.1 Policies for Minority Groups

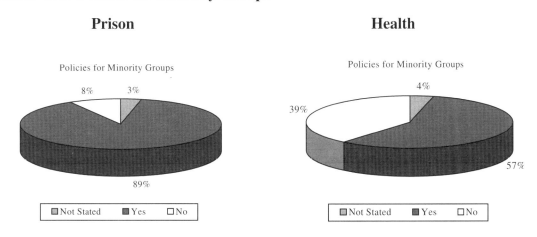

Rassool (1995) reports that approximately 6% of the total population (about 3 million people) make up the ethnic minorities population of England and Wales, Afro-Caribbean, black African, black other, Asians (Indian, Pakistani and Bangladeshi), Chinese, Arab, and mixed origin.

137

Statistically these groups have a much lower takwe up of general medical services (Rassool 1995). Thismay be due to a multitude of factors, including cultural values systems, cultural dissonance, education and literacy, previous experience of persecution, communication difficulties, religious and cultural prescriptions and discrimination.

England's Chief Medical Officer's report (Calman 1992) stated that in order to meet the health needs of its local population a health authority's first requirement is to obtain accurate information about its' ethnic mix. Epidemiological evidence showed that ethno-cultural groups are at greater risk in respect of most of the key areas identified in the White Paper (Department of Health 1992).

It is well established that mortality from coronary heart disease is higher in people from the Indian subcontinent and African Commonwealth; mortality from stroke is higher in Caribbean's, Asians and Africans; and mortality from hypertension is also higher in these ethnic groups than the indigenous population (Balajaran 1991, Marmot *et al.* 1984, Donaldson & Taylor 1983, Cruikshank *et al.* 1980).

Young Asian women have been reported to have a higher rate of suicide and attempted suicide, than other groups. There are also somatic health issues, namely diabetes, sickle cell disorder, thalassaemia and high perinatal mortality which are racial/genetic-specific, affecting particular groups.

People from different cultures are also more likely than whites to be from deprived backgrounds, and may be further disadvantaged by religious/cultural differences and language barriers, and also have to endure racism: both institutional and individual.

To address these issues, Watson (1990) suggests that health-care resources must be offered in a more accessible and acceptable way to people from the ethnic minorities if uptake by the more reticent groups is to improve

Research is needed to ascertain whether nurses feel they are equipped to identify and meet the health-care needs of ethnic minority patients and whether nurses' and patients' expectations of health-care services are similar and indeed compatible.

"Through education, nurses should be able to learn about the values, customs and traditions of different cultures. We must, however, be alert to the dangers of cultural stereotyping. As nurses, we must always remember that our patients are individuals." (Watson 1990)

Nurse education has yet to meet the challenge of preparing practitioners to deliver effective and appropriate health care which meets the needs of minority ethnic groups. The research of Papadopoulos & Alleyne (1995) identified five major categories relevant to nurses caring for ethnic minority clients:

- communication
- nurse-client relationship
- relatives
- nurses' feelings of frustration, stress and helplessness
- lack of knowledge.

Black & Laws (1986) that nurses and doctors often exhibit negative attitudes towards ethnic minority clients have also identified it.

Infection control in prisons and hospitals in the UK

The increase in HIV and hepatitis infections has led to an increased need to control the risk of infection particularly among intravenous drug users. The risk of infection generally follows from needle and syringe sharing, although intoxication with any drugs, including alcohol, may increase risk if only by impairing judgement. To reduce the risk, processes have been in place for a number of years. Cole and Taylor (1999) summarise these developments, they cite an annual report from the Chief Medical Officer at the Department of Health who made recommendations on a number of issues in prisons, including communicable diseases (Acheson 1994). He recommended that sodium hypochlorite tablets be made available to prisoners for the sterilisation of syringes and other equipment that might be used for administering drugs, as was already the practice in Scotland. He welcomed the recommendations of the Joint Committee on Vaccination and Immunisation to offer hepatitis B immunisation to all long term and special risk prisoners. He also recommended that condoms be made available for use by prisoners in England and Wales. Almost simultaneously, the AIDS Advisory Committee to the Home Office made similar recommendations. The recommendations on substance misuse were implemented in September 1995.

Cole and Taylor (1999) report that in hospitals, infection control officers and committees were appointed in all acute hospitals in 1959. This followed pandemic staphylococcal infections in the 1950s. An outbreak of salmonella poisoning at the Stanley Royd Hospital in 1984, and the subsequent report, ensured the extension of such services to long stay hospitals, including the Special Hospitals. By November 1986 there had been the first meeting of an infection control committee in Broadmoor, and by 1988 the committee and its work was similar to that to be found in any NHS hospital. It included external specialist representation, and a full time infection control nurse was appointed for the hospital. One of the earliest tasks of the committee was to formulate a policy on HIV and AIDS. It quickly produced a fact sheet for the staff.

Findings

In the majority of cases the services to meet physical health needs provided tend to be on a needs led basis rather than on a preventative basis. The physical healthcare needs of patients, both within the health care and prison sectors are met in a number of ways according to the institutional processes these include:

- access to full GP services
- specialist consultants providing sessional clinics
- in house provision from Senior House Officers and Registrars
- Well Woman/Man Clinics
- health promotion/education activities and awareness raising
- referrals to local NHS hospitals.

Results from the audits carried out (nine in the health sector and nine in the criminal justice system) were examined together with details from the focused interviews, focus groups and comments from the 115 organisational questionnaires in relation to physical health care. From this analysis it was possible to identify five key themes including environmental issues, lifestyle, and major health demands, management problems and education issues.

Environmental Issues

A frequent problem mentioned related to the poor state of accommodation available in which to provide care. This created specific problems particularly in relation to aspects such as privacy, when invasive procedures proved to be necessary. In comparison to a general medical ward in a general hospital resources were often poor and nurses were called upon to fulfil a multiplicity of roles. Notably, in the prison system, in the absence of support such as pharmacy there were clear dilemmas in relation to dispensing medication. The poor design and layout of accommodation created observation difficulties and nurses had to be creative in overcoming the security and physical health demands of people in their care.

Within the health sector, caring for physical ailments in secure environments presented with different problems. Smaller units do not have the luxury of dedicated wards in which to care for physically ill people and are therefore forced to accommodate ill or recovering individuals alongside an otherwise physically well population. It was often the case that general hospitals were keen to move the person on, but this often meant a quite ill or incapacitated individual having to be housed in less than ideal circumstances.

The problems in relation to accommodation were also matched with paucity in relation to facilities. One extreme example was a secure environment where dental treatment was conducted under general anaesthetic with no provision for recovery. Consequently, patients were often expected to return to their wards in a confused state, with the nursing staff managing the best they could to support the individual.

Most of the services relied on contracts with local general practitioner services and nursing staff felt that in general these were satisfactory. Some services continue to employ their own medical staff for physical health care, particularly in the prison service. In these circumstances it was felt that standards were more variable. In the audits conducted in response to the criteria: "In the event physical ill-health, patients have access to a GP", four of the eighteen services were unable to respond positively to this, which clearly gives some concern about the level and standard of medical care available.

A number of secure environments have looked to contracts for specialist medical care on site, in addition to that of primary health care or general practice. For example a contract has been developed between a secure environment and a local trust for sessions from a consultant surgeon. He is called upon to perform a number of key tasks including complex suturing. These are often cases, mainly women, who have repeatedly cut themselves and have reopened scar tissue. It is felt contracts such as these can be both cost-effective and less of a risk to security as patients do not have to be escorted off the premises.

Policies in relation to physical health were found to be variable in standard, availability and implementation. It was notable that some sites had adopted known national policies. For example, the Scottish Prison Service have adapted the Marsden Clinical Handbook on physical care, as its Clinical Nursing Guidelines, an approach also taken by Ashworth Hospital Authority in Merseyside.

While there is much to commend this approach for its expediency and access to evidence based policies, care will need to be taken that the environment can support the policies in relation to facilities and nursing skills in conducting tasks. The provision of policies is only part of the solution, albeit an important one.

As in all aspects of secure health care, teamwork and support to nursing staff was seen to be of paramount importance. In practice it was patchy and uncoordinated.

Lifestyles

Many nurses stressed the need for empathic understanding when working in the health centres, as they were regularly confronted with individuals where judgements were easy particular in relation to self- injury. Once again, training was highlighted as a key need and was not routinely available on updating physical nursing skills.

Many nurses commented on the lifestyles pursued by many patients before their admission to secure care, which did not lend itself to either good mental or physical health. They described how some individuals could be admitted in a very dishevelled state and without regular access to health care when living in the community; that was particularly true for those that had been sleeping rough before arrest or admission.

The high number of individuals with a history of abuse was a dynamic which appeared to manifest itself in expression by means of self injury and violence. Many patients had a history of abusing a wide range of drugs and substances as well as routine alcohol abuse which for many had taken its toll physically.

The sedentary lifestyle pursued by a number of patients, combined with low income, a poor diet and the consequential problems of obesity was commented upon. A very high number of patients in both the Health and prison sector were heavy smokers. This profile of individuals led to higher instances of health demands when compared with a similar age band of population in the community.

It has been claimed that the health care service for prisoners provides quicker access both to primary and specialist care than the NHS, and all prescriptions are free. (Reed and Lyne 1997) Some nursing staff, particularly in the prison service felt that the level and access to health care was far superior to that enjoyed by people in the community. This was felt to be particularly so in relation to waiting times for surgery or out patient appointments. The impression gained from this comment was an attitude from some staff that patients in these environments were less worthy of what was regarded as preferential treatment. This view may belie a more general underlying attitude to the patient population as a whole

Major Health Demands

The major health demands reported from both sectors included asthma, diabetes, epilepsy and genito-urinary conditions. In keeping with this, particularly within the prison service, these were the most frequently found protocols and examples were available of these being produced at a national level. However, when auditing the eighteen services we inquired whether advice and/or clinics were provided on issues such as asthma and diabetes, these were not available in 3 of the 18 services audited, 2 from the Prison service and 1 from Health.

Issues regarding infection control featured highly in nursing staffs' concern, particularly in relation to Hepatitis A, B and C and also HIV issues. Nurses had a high level of awareness with regard to these issues but concern remained that resources and facilities were sometimes inadequate to meet demand. There was a particular concern over the low availability of counselling services for HIV positive patients.

Given the predominantly young population that both sectors are dealing with, and in particular the prison service, soft tissue injuries as a consequence of sports injuries or fights were commonly seen and treated within the health centre. As well as needing practice nurse skills it was felt that some skills in relation to responding to minor injuries would be useful particularly in the criminal justice system.

There were some examples cited of preventative work, particularly in relation to screening for testicular, cervical and breast cancer, sexual health and the availability of dentists and opticians. The audits examined specific issues in this area and in response to whether there was an identifiable health promotion nurse six of the eighteen services audited were unable to identify such an individual. The services were reviewed for the availability of monthly health checks at ward level, including blood pressure, urinalysis, pulse and weight. Only five of the eighteen services were able to meet this criteria. Furthermore, when the availability of annual dental check-ups was examined six of the eighteen services were also unable to meet this criteria.

Specific problems were highlighted from the women's services visited in the criminal justice system with regard to pregnancy, babies and children. Some very positive work has occurred in this area in recent years, most notably at Styal and Holloway prisons, it was still felt however that additional work was necessary, particularly in relation to the implementation and monitoring of standards.

Management Problems

Nursing staff identified a number of management problems regarding physical health care. For many in the prison service there was a problem in relation to access particularly when people remained in the prison wings rather than in the health centres. Security procedures are such that to have direct contact with individuals when the prisons were on patrol status is almost impossible, this clearly had serious implications in relation to assessment and continuity of care and therapies.

Confidentiality was raised as a major problem, particularly within the criminal justice system and had serious implications in relation to managing individuals with HIV infection in particular. A major dilemma for nurses was when situations arose in which the commitment to confidentiality was tested. They would be put under severe pressure from prison officers and governor grades to release confidential health information concerning individuals because this clearly had implications for the management of the individual in the wider prison setting. Nurses working in prison regard this as a major issue and felt that clarification was necessary within the service to protect their position.

Consent to treatment was seen as particularly difficult in relation to mental health problems. A health centre in a prison is not designated as a place for treatment under the Mental Health Acts, therefore, treatments cannot be administered without the patient's co-operation and consent. This is often frustrating and exasperating for staff, as in the absence of consent they have to await a transfer to NHS centres so that treatment may commence. Prison nurses hope that the current review of the Mental Health Acts might help to resolve some of these issues. The issue of consent also impacts on practice in relation to physical health care in issues such as self- injury, where surgery may be indicated after objects have been ingested (a problem for both the health and criminal justice sectors) and also difficulties surrounding anorexia.

Problems in relation to self-harm, are increasingly becoming apparent amongst the male population, this is usually associated with a personality disorder, and there is a clear statistical link between self- harm and suicide. Prisoners are often transferred into health centres during acute suicide risk for increased observation. In the health sector, examples of serious self-mutilation by psychotic patients have not been uncommon and has created enormous demands on observation time and ethical problems in relation to restraint.

Linking with families and friends of patients in the Prison Services, particularly of those inmates that remain in health centres for some time, is acknowledged as a limitation. This was also a problem in some parts of the secure health sector, that continued to have centralised visiting. Nurses including primary nurses expressed frustration about the limited amount of contact they had with patients families.

Some comment was made in relation to language problems, and the growing number of ethnic minority groups were over represented in both the prison and health sector. When auditing services, we examined whether interpretation services were available if required and were disappointed to find that in four of the eighteen services audited this was not routinely available.

Another key problem for secure environments is the requirement for individuals to attend for emergency or outpatient appointments in the wider NHS. This is a clear problem in relation to a risk to security and is one in particular where services have been criticised for being over zealous in the application of security measure such as handcuffs. This is perhaps an example where the therapy security dichotomy is brought into sharp relief and accentuated. One way that some secure environments have attempted to minimise this risk is by increasing the amount of physical health care provided within in their own services.

Education Issues

The final theme that emerged from the qualitative analysis related to education issues in relation to the patient population. This was accentuated in the audits where it was found that little or no information was displayed on notice boards or made generally available to patients.

Patients in Secure NHS provision tend to present with severe or enduring mental illness or learning disability. This can result in long term neglect, which when combined with a sedentary lifestyle, high levels of smoking and long term reliance on medication which many patients experience, increases the risk of physical illnesses occurring. A significant proportion of the Prison population presents with similar problems and utilises the health care services to a great extent. Many of these issues are being addressed through Health Promotion programmes targeted at specific needs such as smoking, healthy eating and well man/woman clinics. Written advice to patients regarding medication side effects and contra-indications was poor and in the main non-existent. The availability of advice to patients on health care issues including health promotion could be improved, although some examples of good practice were identified.

It was felt there was a greater skill deficit in the health care sector in relation to physical health care. Often meeting patients physical health needs in these predominantly psychiatric services was often seen as an afterthought and provided little evidence of a systematic and co-ordinated approach to this aspect of care. Clearly this whole issue raises both organisational and training implications in order to improve practice in both sectors.

Conclusions

Key informants and focus groups provided information about some of the particular issues with regard to care of the physical health care needs of the three key groups identified; women, pregnant women and people from different cultural backgrounds. The following issues were identified:

- Patients in secure settings have particular physical health care needs, which are related to their pre-existing vulnerabilities, level of competency, co-morbidity and mental disorders.

- Identification of these needs by practitioners is complicated by the behavioural and personality characteristics, which either exacerbate expressed symptoms and demands or prevent their identification.

- Environment, lifestyle, health demands, managerial and educational issues are identified as major concerns in relation to the provision of physical health care in all secure settings.

- The issue of pregnant women and women with children in prisons poses particular ethical and practical difficulties for nurses and midwives. Action has been taken in some organisations that could be applied more widely.

- Patients from ethnic minority groups have relatively poor levels of health and their needs often go unrecognised. Services provided to these groups should be the subject of further evaluation and development

- Infection control is an issue that pre-dominates, particularly within Prisons, and nurses need to remain up-dated on developments in this area.

Project Leader

Les Storey, Senior Lecturer, Faculty of Health, University of Central Lancashire

Colin Dale (joint Project Leader from July 1998 to January 1999)

Steering Group

Hamza Aumeer, English National Board,

Lindsay Bates, Prison Service, England and Wales, (from April 1999)

Martin Bradley, Council Member

Patrick Keavney, Council Member

Tony Leslie, Scottish Prison Service (from January 1999)

Paul Lewis, Council Member

Brodie Paterson, Senior Lecturer, Stirling University

Barry Topping-Morris, Head of Nursing, Caswell Clinic

Yvonne Willmott, Prison Service, England and Wales, July 1998, December 1998

Rosaleen Malone, Council Member, July 1998- September 1998

Richard Bradshaw, Professional Officer, Mental Health and Learning Disabilities, UKCC

External Reviewers

Dr Colin Holmes, Professor of Nursing (Mental Health) University of Western Sydney

Dr Kevin Powers, Professor of Clinical Psychology, University of Stirling

Acknowledgements

Research/Administrative Staff

Anneke Constable

Danielle Godwin

Janine Huston

Rachel Ralphson

Project Support Group

Ann Alty, University of Central Lancashire

Peter Green, Mental Health Act Commission

Jennifer Harris, University of Central Lancashire

Paul Tarbuck, Mental Health Services of Salford

Kellie Sherlock, University of Central Lancashire

Special thanks goes to all the nurses and midwives across the UK who participated in the Scoping Exercise, and particularly the following people:

Joe Hilman, Nursing Officer, Department of Health and Social Services, Northern Ireland

Maggi Lyne, Nurse Advisor, HM Inspectorate of Prisons, England and Wales

Sally Newton, Head of Nursing, Northern Ireland Prison Service

Malcolm Rae, Nursing Officer Department of Health

Robert Samuels, Nursing Officer, Scottish Office

Mike Tonkin, Nursing Officer, Welsh Office

Phil Woods, University of Manchester

and the following staff from the University of Central Lancashire

Maureen Dow, Library Assistant, Ormskirk Campus

John Howard, Health Informatics, Post Graduate Medical Centre

Demography
of
Staff Questionnaire Respondents

Job Titles

Job Titles of Prison Service Respondents

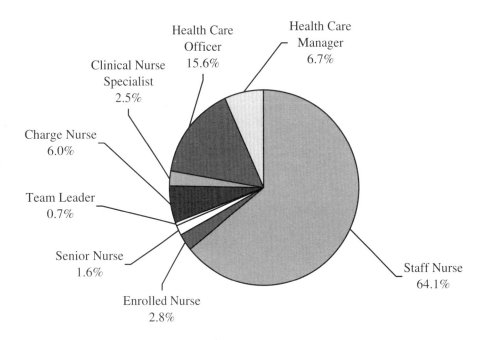

Health Care Officer 15.6%

Health Care Manager 6.7%

Clinical Nurse Specialist 2.5%

Charge Nurse 6.0%

Team Leader 0.7%

Senior Nurse 1.6%

Enrolled Nurse 2.8%

Staff Nurse 64.1%

Job Titles of Health Respondents

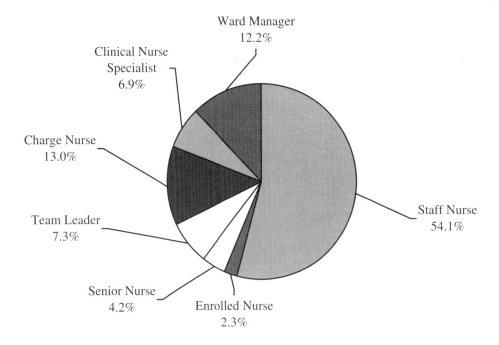

Ward Manager 12.2%

Clinical Nurse Specialist 6.9%

Charge Nurse 13.0%

Team Leader 7.3%

Senior Nurse 4.2%

Enrolled Nurse 2.3%

Staff Nurse 54.1%

148

Job Grades

Job Grades of Prison Service Respondents

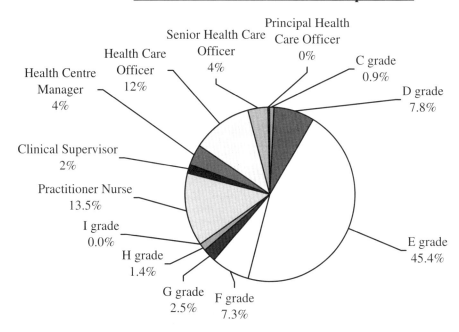

Principal Health Care Officer 0%
Senior Health Care Officer 4%
Health Care Officer 12%
Health Centre Manager 4%
Clinical Supervisor 2%
Practitioner Nurse 13.5%
I grade 0.0%
H grade 1.4%
G grade 2.5%
F grade 7.3%
E grade 45.4%
D grade 7.8%
C grade 0.9%

Job Grades of Health Sector Respondents

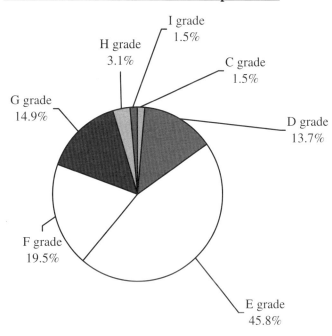

I grade 1.5%
H grade 3.1%
G grade 14.9%
F grade 19.5%
E grade 45.8%
D grade 13.7%
C grade 1.5%

Country Worked In

	England	Scotland	Wales	Northern Ireland
Prison Service	326	90	12	12
Health Care	229	11	27	0 *

* No Health Centre staff were recipients of staff questionnaires. Focus groups and focus interviews were held across the province.

Age Band of respondents

Prison Service Respondents

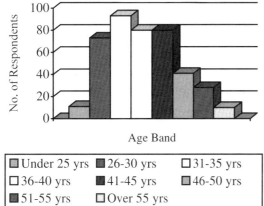

- ☐ Under 25 yrs ■ 26-30 yrs ☐ 31-35 yrs
- ☐ 36-40 yrs ■ 41-45 yrs ■ 46-50 yrs
- ■ 51-55 yrs ☐ Over 55 yrs

Health Sector Respondents

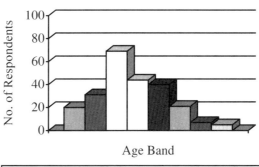

- ☐ Under 25 yrs ■ 26-30 yrs ☐ 31-35 yrs
- ☐ 36-40 yrs ■ 41-45 yrs ■ 46-50 yrs
- ■ 51-55 yrs ☐ Over 55 yrs

Years Qualified

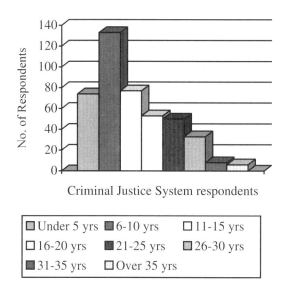

Criminal Justice System respondents

☐ Under 5 yrs	■ 6-10 yrs	☐ 11-15 yrs
☐ 16-20 yrs	■ 21-25 yrs	■ 26-30 yrs
■ 31-35 yrs	☐ Over 35 yrs	

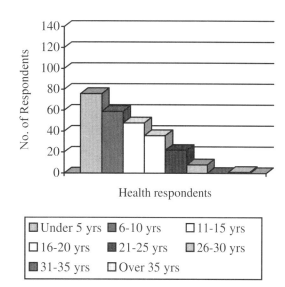

Health respondents

☐ Under 5 yrs	■ 6-10 yrs	☐ 11-15 yrs
☐ 16-20 yrs	■ 21-25 yrs	■ 26-30 yrs
■ 31-35 yrs	☐ Over 35 yrs	

Years Worked In Secure Environments

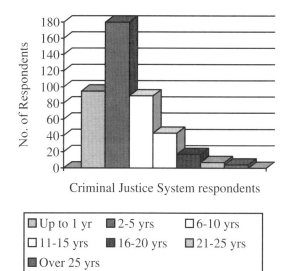

Criminal Justice System respondents

☐ Up to 1 yr	■ 2-5 yrs	☐ 6-10 yrs
☐ 11-15 yrs	■ 16-20 yrs	■ 21-25 yrs
■ Over 25 yrs		

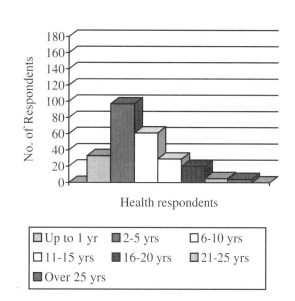

Health respondents

☐ Up to 1 yr	■ 2-5 yrs	☐ 6-10 yrs
☐ 11-15 yrs	■ 16-20 yrs	■ 21-25 yrs
■ Over 25 yrs		

APPENDIX 5.2

Individuals Interviewed during Scoping Exercise

Focused Interviews:

Joe Hilman, Nursing Officer, Department of Health and Social Services, Northern Ireland
Robert Samuels, Nursing Officer, Scottish Office
Mike Tomkin, Nursing Officer, Welsh Office
Malcolm Rae, Nursing Officer Department of Health

Seamus Sloan, National Board for Northern Ireland
Hamza Aumeer, English National Board
Mick Fisher, Welsh National Board
Ian Murray, National Board for Scotland

Yvonne Willmott, Nursing Advisor, Prison Service England and Wales
Sally Newton, Head of Prison Nursing, Northern Ireland
Tony Leslie, Head of Prison Nursing, Scotland
Brian Caton, Prison Officers Association
Ann Norman, RCN Nurses working in prison Forum

Maggi Lyne, Nurse Advisor, HM Inspectorate of Prisons
Chris Tchaikovsky, Women In Prisons
Beverley Beech, Association for Improvement in Maternity Services
Laila Namdarkhan, Women in Special Hospitals

Kevin Gournay, Professor of Nursing, Institute of Psychiatry
Phil Barker, Professor of Psychiatric Nursing, University of Newcastle
David Robinson, Associate Professor of Nursing, Rampton Hospital/ Sheffield University
Sheila Kitzinger, Professor, Wolfson Institute, Thames Valley University

Barry Topping Morris, Head of Nursing, Caswell Clinic, Bridgend
Nigel Maguire, Director of Mental Health, Hutton Centre, Middlesborough (former Executive Nurse, State Hospital Carstairs)
Alan Stirling, Senior Nurse, Broadmoor
Nicola Mahoud, Senior Nurse, Mental Health Services of Salford
Joe Cutler, Professional Development Nurse, Raeside Clinic
Steve Kirby, Lecturer Practitioner, Hutton Centre, Middlesborough
Ian Fidler, Senior Nurse, Rampton
Richard Idle, Ward Manager, Rampton
Barbara Wilson, Senior Nurse Manager, Carstairs
Carol Watson, Professional Development Nurse,
Caroline Wilkinson, Health Care Manager, Usk Prison
Jimmy Noak, Team Leader, Broadmoor Hospital
Ann Aiyegbusi, Nurse Consultant, Ashworth Hospital
Stephanie Dulson, Health Care Manager, Styal Prison

APPENDIX 5.3

Sites Where Focus Groups Were Held

Focus Groups have been conducted in the following locations:

England

Broadmoor	Rampton	Ashworth
Raeside Clinic	Hutton Centre	St Nicholas's Hospital
Ormskirk DGH	UKCC	Abel House
Winchester Prison		

Wales

Welsh National Board	Caswell Clinic	Parc Prison

.

Scotland

Edinburgh Prison	Woodilee Hospital	State Hospital Carstairs

Northern Ireland

Maghabery Prison	Eastern Health and Social Services Board
St Lukes Hospital Armagh	Western Health and Social Services Board

APPENDIX 5.4

**Organisations Contributing
to the
Focus Groups and Audits**

Organisations who contributed to Focus Groups or Audits:

Health Service:

Ashworth
Bethlem Royal Hospital
Broadland Clinic
Broadmoor,
Burston House
Calderstones
Camlet Lodge
Carstairs,
Chadwick Lodge
Downshire, Downpatrick
Edenfield Unit, Salford
Eastern Health and Social
Services Board
Gardner Unit, Salford
Gransha, Londonderry
Hadley Lodge
Holywell
Hutton Centre
John Howard Centre

Kemple View
Kenneth Day Unit
Kestrel Unit
Kneesworth House
Kolvin Unit
Langdale Unit
Marlborough House
Maudsley Hospital
Muckamore
Northern Health and Social
Services Board
Norvic Clinic
Purdysburn
Rampton
Rathbone Hospital, Liverpool
Reaside Clinic
Rowan Unit
Roycroft Unit
Runwell Hospital

Scott Clinic
Scott House
Southern Health and Social
Services Board
St Georges Hospital,
Newcastle
St Lukes, Armagh
St Nicholas Hospital,
Newcastle
Stockton Hall
Tameside General
The Spinney
Trevor Gibbens Unit
Wallingford Clinic
Western Health and Social
Services Board
Woodilee Hospital
Glasgow

Prison Services:

Aberdeen
Aldington
Altcourse
Belmarsh
Buckley Hall
Cookham Wood
Cornton Vale
Dumfries
East Sutton Park
Edinburgh
Elmley
Glenochil
Glen Parva
Greenock

High Down
Holloway
Hydebank Wood
Kirkham
Lancaster Castle
Lancaster Farms
Leicester
Liverpool
Longriggend
Low Moss
Maghabery
Magilligan
Maidstone
Manchester

Maze
Parc
Pentonville
Perth
Polmont
Prescoed
Shots
Standford Hill
Styal
Usk
Wandsworth
Winchester
Wormwood Scrubs

157

Competence Data and Chi Square analysis
from
Staff Questionnaires

Identify the level of involvement that you have within your work role for each of the following nursing interventions:

Legend 1:

			Nursing Intervention		How important are these interventions for nursing in secure environments?					
0	**1**	**2**	**3**	**4**	**0**	**1**	**2**	**3**	**4**	**5**
Not Given	Part of role & Ensure others undertake this	Ensuring others undertake this	Part of role	Not Part of role	Issue	Not Given	Very unimportant	Unimportant	Undecided	Important	Very important

Legend 2:

Example:

67.0
58.0

Health = % of responses from Health Service Nurses

Prison = % of responses from Nurses working in prison

This means that 67% of the Health sample and 58% of the Prison sample responded in this way.

Section 1 - Promote and implement principles which underpin effective, quality and practice

	Nursing Intervention	0	1	2	3	4	How important are these interventions for nursing in secure environments?	0	1	2	3	4	5
Q1.	Promote people's equality, diversity and rights	2.1	33.6	11.0	52.3	1.1		1.4	5.7	0.0	0.4	23.3	69.3
		1.2	14.2	11.8	68.9	3.9		1.6	5.6	1.6	3.2	35.7	52.2
Q2.	Promote effective communication and relationships	2.5	34.3	11.3	51.2	0.7		1.8	6.4	0.0	0.0	14.8	77.0
		1.4	13.9	10.2	71.9	2.6		1.4	5.8	0.7	0.7	25.3	66.1
Q3.	Promote communication with individuals where there are communication differences	3.2	31.4	10.6	53.7	1.1		2.5	5.3	0.0	0.4	19.1	72.8
		1.4	13.9	9.7	69.8	5.1		1.6	5.3	0.5	1.6	29.2	61.7

Section 2 (a) - Assess, develop, implement and improve programmes of care for individuals

0	1	2	3	4	Nursing Intervention	How important are these interventions for nursing in secure environments?					
						0	1	2	3	4	5
2.5	27.2	12.4	57.2	0.7	**Q4.** Assess individuals to determine their overall needs and risk	1.4	6.0	0.0	0.0	11.7	80.9
0.7	10.4	11.8	74.7	2.3		1.9	6.3	0.5	0.2	26.2	65.0
3.9	21.2	9.9	42.8	22.3	**Q5.** Provide specialist assessment services on individuals' needs so that others can take action	6.7	5.7	0.4	3.2	25.8	58.3
1.9	8.6	12.8	61.0	15.8		6.0	4.2	0.5	4.2	32.9	52.2
2.8	25.8	12.7	58.3	0.4	**Q6.** Assist in the assessment of, and the planning of programmes of care for, individuals	1.4	5.7	0.4	0.4	19.1	73.1
1.6	11.4	9.3	74.9	2.8		2.1	5.3	1.2	1.6	36.7	53.1
2.5	27.6	11.7	54.1	4.2	**Q7.** Plan specific therapeutic interventions to enable individuals to recognise and address any socially-unacceptable behaviour	1.1	5.7	0.4	0.4	22.6	70.0
1.9	9.3	10.2	55.2	23.4		8.4	4.9	1.4	6.5	29.0	49.9
2.5	27.2	10.6	59.4	0.4	**Q8.** Contribute to the joint implementation and monitoring of programmes of care for individuals	1.4	5.7	0.4	0.7	20.8	71.0
1.6	9.7	9.0	74.7	4.9		3.0	4.9	0.4	3.5	37.1	51.3
1.8	27.9	12.4	54.4	3.5	**Q9.** Implement specific therapeutic interventions to enable individuals to manage their behaviour	0.7	4.6	0.4	1.4	26.9	66.1
1.2	8.4	10.9	53.6	26.0		9.5	4.2	0.5	5.8	38.5	41.5
2.1	25.8	11.7	56.0	2.5	**Q10.** Assist in the implementation and monitoring of specific therapeutic interventions	2.1	4.6	0.4	1.1	30.4	61.5
1.4	7.7	8.4	64.7	17.9		8.1	3.7	0.7	6.3	42.7	38.5
2.1	26.9	13.1	55.5	2.5	**Q11.** Enable individuals to develop and maintain skills of independent living	2.1	4.2	1.4	2.1	28.6	61.5
2.1	7.4	8.4	58.0	24.1		8.4	3.7	1.4	7.9	37.1	41.5
3.2	27.2	8.8	57.6	3.2	**Q12.** Enable individuals to develop meaningful relationships with others	2.1	3.9	1.1	4.9	32.9	55.1
2.3	6.7	8.6	53.8	28.5		11.6	3.7	2.2	10.7	38.1	33.6
2.1	29.3	8.1	57.2	3.1	**Q13.** Enable individuals who are at risk to themselves and others to identify behavioural boundaries and develop control	1.1	4.9	0.4	2.1	18.7	72.8
2.1	9.3	10.9	66.6	11.1		5.3	4.4	0.5	2.8	33.4	53.6

Section 2 (b) - Assess, develop, implement and improve programmes of care for individuals

0	1	2	3	4	Nursing Intervention	How important are these interventions for nursing in secure environments?					
						0	1	2	3	4	5
2.1	25.1	9.2	63.3	0.4	Q14. Contribute to the evaluation and improvement of	1.4	4.6	0.4	1.1	28.6	64.0
2.3	9.0	9.3	73.8	5.6	programmes of care for individuals	3.9	4.2	0.2	2.6	41.1	48.0
3.5	18.4	10.6	50.2	17.3	Q15. Assess individuals' needs for primary health care services	5.7	4.2	1.1	7.8	35.33	45.9
0.9	8.1	8.8	72.6	9.5		5.1	4.2	0.9	3.7	38.1	48.0
4.9	15.2	10.6	44.9	24.4	Q16. Develop, monitor and review programmes of primary	8.8	4.9	1.4	9.5	31.1	44.2
1.2	7.2	7.7	68.7	15.3	health care for individuals	5.6	4.2	0.9	5.1	42.2	42.0
3.2	22.3	9.9	61.5	3.2	Q17. Contribute to raising awareness of health issues	1.8	4.2	1.1	4.6	39.9	48.4
1.4	10.2	8.8	76.3	3.2		2.8	3.9	0.5	2.6	37.1	53.1
2.1	23.7	8.8	63.6	1.8	Q18. Enable individuals to address issues which affect their	1.4	4.6	0.7	2.8	38.2	52.3
0.9	7.9	10.4	78.9	1.9	health and well-being	2.1	3.9	0.9	1.6	39.7	51.7
3.2	17.0	8.5	47.3	24.0	Q19. Raise awareness of the needs of individuals discharged	8.1	5.3	0.7	4.9	27.2	53.7
3.2	7.0	9.7	56.1	23.9	from your services	8.8	3.9	1.2	8.1	37.4	40.6
4.2	13.1	5.7	27.9	49.1	Q20. Promote the needs of individuals in the community	15.5	3.9	2.5	12.4	22.6	43.1
2.6	3.9	8.1	28.5	56.8		22.5	3.9	3.7	13.0	30.2	26.7
3.9	13.8	6.0	38.9	37.5	Q21. Negotiate, agree and support placements for individuals	11.3	3.9	2.5	9.9	24.4	48.1
2.6	4.2	5.8	30.6	56.8		21.8	3.9	3.0	14.4	30.4	26.5
3.9	15.2	6.4	38.2	36.4	Q22. Develop, monitor and review discharge packages to	11.3	3.2	2.5	9.2	24.4	49.5
2.8	5.6	7.7	31.8	52.2	manage individuals	20.0	3.7	3.0	11.1	31.8	30.4

Section 3 - Create and maintain environments and relationships with individuals which value them as people and support their therapeutic goals

0	1	2	3	4	Nursing Intervention	How important are these interventions for nursing in secure environments?					
						0	1	2	3	4	5
3.9	24.7	7.8	54.8	8.8	**Q23.** Contribute to the provision of effective physical, social and emotional environments for group care	4.9	3.5	0.7	3.4	33.6	54.1
3.9	6.0	7.4	53.6	29.0		15.1	3.7	1.9	9.0	41.5	28.8
3.2	26.1	6.7	62.2	1.8	**Q24.** Build and sustain relationships with individuals to reinforce their therapeutic goals	2.5	4.2	0.7	0.4	26.1	66.1
2.8	6.7	7.4	72.2	10.9		8.4	3.5	0.9	5.8	44.1	37.4
3.5	27.6	4.2	61.8	2.8	**Q25.** Physically intervene in situations where there is a breakdown in environments and relationships to limit risks to those involved	2.5	4.2	0.7	1.8	26.5	64.3
3.0	7.2	6.3	56.8	26.7		11.8	3.5	1.2	10.2	37.4	36.0
4.2	25.1	5.3	61.1	4.2	**Q26.** Support individuals with difficult or potentially difficult relationships	3.2	3.5	0.7	2.1	35.0	55.5
3.9	7.7	6.7	70.8	10.9		7.9	3.5	0.5	7.2	45.5	35.5
4.6	22.3	7.4	60.1	5.7	**Q27.** Enable individuals to maintain contacts in isolating situations	4.2	3.2	0.7	2.5	33.6	55.8
2.6	6.5	6.0	61.3	23.7		10.9	4.4	0.9	9.0	40.6	34.1
5.3	21.2	6.4	60.1	7.1	**Q28.** Enable individuals to adjust to and manage their loss	6.0	3.2	1.1	3.9	31.1	54.8
3.9	6.7	6.3	70.3	12.8		9.5	3.5	0.9	6.7	42.2	37.1
4.9	16.3	8.1	50.2	20.5	**Q29.** Enable individuals' partners, relatives and friends to adjust to and manage the individual's loss	7.4	3.5	1.8	7.1	35.3	44.9
3.5	3.2	4.6	26.0	62.6		27.1	3.9	4.2	17.4	25.8	21.6
3.9	17.3	8.8	51.2	18.7	**Q30.** Enable individuals, their partners, relatives and friends to explore and manage change	6.7	3.9	1.8	6.4	36.0	45.2
4.2	3.7	3.9	31.3	56.8		26.0	3.2	3.9	17.2	26.9	22.7
5.7	13.8	6.7	34.3	39.6	**Q31.** Contribute to establishing and running mutual support networks	13.8	3.9	1.8	14.1	26.1	40.3
3.2	3.5	5.1	38.1	50.1		21.1	4.2	4.6	13.0	30.9	26.2
3.2	27.2	5.7	62.9	1.1	**Q32.** Support individuals when they are distressed	1.8	4.2	0.0	1.1	27.9	65.0
2.1	9.3	7.0	79.1	2.6		3.6	4.9	0.2	1.2	33.9	57.3
6.0	20.1	4.6	47.3	21.9	**Q33.** Create and maintain boundaries between the community and individuals detained in secure conditions	10.2	4.6	0.7	11.0	25.8	47.7
3.9	5.6	5.6	38.5	46.4		24.4	4.2	3.7	10.4	27.4	29.9
3.9	29.0	5.2	59.4	2.5	**Q34.** Protect patients from themselves and each other	2.5	4.2	0.7	1.8	26.1	64.7
2.1	9.7	7.2	71.5	9.5		6.3	4.6	0.2	3.0	31.3	54.5

	0	1	2	3	4		0	1	2	3	4	5
Q35. Contribute to the protection of individuals from abuse	4.2	29.3	6.7	57.6	2.1		2.5	4.2	0.0	0.7	23.7	68.9
	1.9	9.7	6.7	74.2	7.4			6.5	4.2	0.2	2.1	33.4	53.6
Q36. Escort patients within and beyond secure settings	3.5	27.9	7.8	56.2	4.6		2.1	3.9	0.4	4.2	24.4	65.0
	2.3	5.6	5.8	42.0	44.3			18.6	5.1	4.2	10.7	30.2	31.3

Section 4 - Provide and improve resources and services which facilitate organisational functioning

Nursing Intervention	0	1	2	3	4		How important are these interventions for nursing in secure environments?					
							0	1	2	3	4	5
Q37. Manage one's caseload against the prioritised needs of individuals.	5.2	17.7	8.8	55.1	13.1		6.7	3.5	1.8	6.7	33.9	47.3
	3.5	7.4	7.7	62.9	18.6		10.9	4.4	1.6	8.6	38.7	35.7
Q38. Support and lead teams to enable work objectives to be met	4.6	14.8	8.1	54.8	17.7		7.1	3.9	1.4	3.5	30.4	53.7
	3.2	7.4	8.4	44.5	36.4		17.9	2.8	0.9	7.2	35.7	35.5
Q39. Support staff in maintaining their identity and safe personal boundaries	3.2	17.3	7.1	65.0	7.4		4.2	3.2	0.7	1.4	25.4	65.0
	3.0	7.9	6.6	58.7	24.1		13.2	3.0	0.5	2.8	34.3	46.2
Q40. Counsel and support staff in times of stress	4.6	14.5	6.4	64.3	10.2		4.2	3.5	0.7	1.4	20.5	69.6
	1.6	7.0	6.0	62.6	22.7		10.4	3.9	0.2	2.8	24.6	58.0
Q41. Promote, monitor and maintain health, safety and security in the workplace	2.5	23.0	6.4	64.7	3.5		3.2	4.2	0.0	0.4	22.6	69.6
	1.9	9.7	6.7	73.3	8.4		3.7	3.9	0.0	2.1	29.2	61.0
Q42. Receive, transmit, store and retrieve information	3.2	25.8	5.7	61.8	3.5		2.8	3.9	0.0	2.5	27.2	63.6
	1.6	9.3	7.4	76.6	5.1		3.0	4.2	0.2	2.3	35.7	54.5

Section 5 - Develop the knowledge, competence and practice of self and others

					Nursing Intervention	How important are these interventions for nursing in secure environments?					
0	1	2	3	4		0	1	2	3	4	5
2.8	23.3	4.6	68.6	0.7	**Q43.** Contribute to the development of knowledge and practice	2.1	4.6	0.0	0.4	26.1	66.8
1.6	9.3	6.3	78.4	4.4		3.0	4.2	0.0	2.3	29.0	61.5
2.5	20.8	4.9	71.0	0.7	**Q44.** Develop oneself within the role	1.4	4.6	0.4	0.7	24.7	68.2
1.4	7.4	6.5	82.8	1.9		2.3	4.6	0.0	0.7	27.8	64.5
2.8	21.9	5.7	65.7	3.9	**Q45.** Contribute to the development of others	2.8	4.2	0.4	0.7	29.0	62.9
1.9	9.0	6.5	73.5	9.0		3.9	4.4	0.0	2.6	30.6	58.5

Chi-square results (health care/prison) between those reporting it to be part of their role and those reporting that it was not (df=1).

Competency	χ^2	N
Q1. Promote people's equality, diversity and rights	4.136 *	703
Q2. Promote effective communication and relationships	2.251	701
Q3. Promote communication with individuals where there are communication differences	6.908 **	699
Q4. Assess individuals to determine their overall needs and risk	1.729	704
Q5. Provide specialist assessment services on individuals' needs so that others can take action	4.981 *	695
Q6. Assist in the assessment of, and the planning of programmes of care for, individuals	4.291 *	699
Q7. Plan specific therapeutic interventions to enable individuals to recognise and address any socially-unacceptable behaviour	45.573 ***	699
Q8. Contribute to the joint implementation and monitoring of programmes of care for individuals	10.114 ***	700
Q9. Implement specific therapeutic interventions to enable individuals to manage their behaviour	58.900 ***	704
Q10. Assist in the implementation and monitoring of specific therapeutic interventions	37.230 ***	702
Q11. Enable individuals to develop and maintain skills of independent living	59.596 ***	699
Q12. Enable individuals to develop meaningful relationships with others	70.866 ***	695
Q13. Enable individuals who are at risk to themselves and others to identify behavioural boundaries and develop control	13.676 ***	699
Q14. Contribute to the evaluation and improvement of programmes of care for individuals	12.291 ***	698
Q15. Assess individuals' needs for primary health care services	9.624 **	700
Q16. Develop, monitor and review programmes of primary health care for individuals	10.230 **	695
Q17. Contribute to raising awareness of health issues	0.000	699
Q18. Enable individuals to address issues which affect their health and well-being	0.000	704
Q19. Raise awareness of the needs of individuals discharged from your services	0.000	691
Q20. Promote the needs of individuals in the community	3.029	691
Q21. Negotiate, agree and support placements for individuals	23.994 ***	692
Q22. Develop, monitor and review discharge packages to manage individuals	15.949 ***	691
Q23. Contribute to the provision of effective physical, social and emotional environments for group care	41.160 ***	686
Q24. Build and sustain relationships with individuals to reinforce their therapeutic goals	19.725 ***	693
Q25. Physically intervene in situations where there is a breakdown in environments and relationships to limit risks to those involved	66.530 ***	691
Q26. Support individuals with difficult or potentially difficult relationships	9.117 **	685
Q27. Enable individuals to maintain contacts in isolating situations	37.793 ***	690
Q28. Enable individuals to adjust to and manage their loss	5.055 *	682
Q29. Enable individuals' partners, relatives and friends to adjust to and manage the individual's loss	121.246 ***	685
Q30. Enable individuals, their partners, relatives and friends to explore and manage change	104.274 ***	685
Q31. Contribute to establishing and running mutual support networks	5.941 *	684
Q32. Support individuals when they are distressed	1.236	696
Q33. Create and maintain boundaries between the community and individuals detained in secure conditions	41.690 ***	680
Q34. Protect patients from themselves and each other	12.019 ***	694
Q35. Contribute to the protection of individuals from abuse	8.133 **	694
Q36. Escort patients within and beyond secure settings	129.623 ***	694

Q37. Manage one's caseload against the prioritised needs of individuals	3.011	684
Q38. Support and lead teams to enable work objectives to be met	27.591 ***	687
Q39. Support staff in maintaining their identity and safe personal boundaries	31.992 ***	692
Q40. Counsel and support staff in times of stress	16.072 ***	694
Q41. Promote, monitor and maintain health, safety and security in the workplace	5.719 *	699
Q42. Receive, transmit, store and retrieve information	0.584	698
Q43. Contribute to the development of knowledge and practice	6.830 **	699
Q44. Develop oneself within the role	0.878	701
Q45. Contribute to the development of others	6.066 *	698

[χ^2 = chi-square incorporating Yates' correction for continuity; * significant (<0.05); ** highly significant (<0.01); * very highly significant (<0.001)]**

Chi-square results (health care/prison) between level of importance reported (df=2).

Competency	χ^2	N
Q1. Promote people's equality, diversity and rights	7.835 *	703
Q2. Promote effective communication and relationships	1.978	703
Q3. Promote communication with individuals where there are communication differences	2.546	700
Q4. Assess individuals to determine their overall needs and risk	0.827	702
Q5. Provide specialist assessment services on individuals' needs so that others can take action	1.079	699
Q6. Assist in the assessment of, and the planning of programmes of care for, individuals	2.627	701
Q7. Plan specific therapeutic interventions to enable individuals to recognise and address any socially-unacceptable behaviour	18.460 ***	675
Q8. Contribute to the joint implementation and monitoring of programmes of care for individuals	5.939	697
Q9. Implement specific therapeutic interventions to enable individuals to manage their behaviour	9.879 **	671
Q10. Assist in the implementation and monitoring of specific therapeutic interventions	12.588 **	673
Q11. Enable individuals to develop and maintain skills of independent living	12.078 **	672
Q12. Enable individuals to develop meaningful relationships with others	10.954 **	658
Q13. Enable individuals who are at risk to themselves and others to identify behavioural boundaries and develop control	0.425	688
Q14. Contribute to the evaluation and improvement of programmes of care for individuals	2.152	693
Q15. Assess individuals' needs for primary health care services	5.778	676
Q16. Develop, monitor and review programmes of primary health care for individuals	6.936 *	665
Q17. Contribute to raising awareness of health issues	2.450	697
Q18. Enable individuals to address issues which affect their health and well-being	1.246	701
Q19. Raise awareness of the needs of individuals discharged from your services	2.938	653
Q20. Promote the needs of individuals in the community	1.629	573
Q21. Negotiate, agree and support placements for individuals	6.971 *	588
Q22. Develop, monitor and review discharge packages to manage individuals	2.839	596
Q23. Contribute to the provision of effective physical, social and emotional environments for group care	13.743 ***	635
Q24. Build and sustain relationships with individuals to reinforce their therapeutic goals	15.531 ***	671
Q25. Physically intervene in situations where there is a breakdown in environments and relationships to limit risks to those involved	22.246 ***	656
Q26. Support individuals with difficult or potentially difficult relationships	9.833 **	671
Q27. Enable individuals to maintain contacts in isolating situations	15.750 ***	655
Q28. Enable individuals to adjust to and manage their loss	3.106	656
Q29. Enable individuals' partners, relatives and friends to adjust to and manage the individual's loss	36.674 ***	576
Q30. Enable individuals, their partners, relatives and friends to explore and manage change	34.570 ***	583
Q31. Contribute to establishing and running mutual support networks	3.700	584
Q32. Support individuals when they are distressed	0.329	698
Q33. Create and maintain boundaries between the community and individuals detained in secure conditions	4.419	580
Q34. Protect patients from themselves and each other	1.272	680
Q35. Contribute to the protection of individuals from abuse	2.411	679
Q36. Escort patients within and beyond secure settings	26.940 ***	628
Q37. Manage one's caseload against the prioritised needs of individuals	1.599	648

164

Q38. Support and lead teams to enable work objectives to be met	6.238 *	617
Q39. Support staff in maintaining their identity and safe personal boundaries	1.950	645
Q40. Counsel and support staff in times of stress	1.822	657
Q41. Promote, monitor and maintain health, safety and security in the workplace	3.771	689
Q42. Receive, transmit, store and retrieve information	0.133	693
Q43. Contribute to the development of knowledge and practice	4.447	695
Q44. Develop oneself within the role	0.026	700
Q45. Contribute to the development of others	3.325	689

[χ^2 = chi-square, * significant (<0.05); ** highly significant (<0.01); *** very highly significant (<0.001)]

Chi-square results comparing high secure and medium secure units for those reporting it to be part of their role those reporting that it was not (df=1).

Competency	χ^2	N
Q1. Promote people's equality, diversity and rights	0.414	208
Q2. Promote effective communication and relationships	0.000	208
Q3. Promote communication with individuals where there are communication differences	0.397	206
Q4. Assess individuals to determine their overall needs and risk	0.000	208
Q5. Provide specialist assessment services on individuals' needs so that others can take action	0.637	205
Q6. Assist in the assessment of, and the planning of programmes of care for, individuals	0.126	207
Q7. Plan specific therapeutic interventions to enable individuals to recognise and address any socially-unacceptable behaviour	0.317	208
Q8. Contribute to the joint implementation and monitoring of programmes of care for individuals	0.011	208
Q9. Implement specific therapeutic interventions to enable individuals to manage their behaviour	0.012	209
Q10. Assist in the implementation and monitoring of specific therapeutic interventions	0.186	208
Q11. Enable individuals to develop and maintain skills of independent living	0.000	209
Q12. Enable individuals to develop meaningful relationships with others	0.000	207
Q13. Enable individuals who are at risk to themselves and others to identify behavioural boundaries and develop control	0.024	209
Q14. Contribute to the evaluation and improvement of programmes of care for individuals	0.137	208
Q15. Assess individuals' needs for primary health care services	2.673	206
Q16. Develop, monitor and review programmes of primary health care for individuals	0.436	203
Q17. Contribute to raising awareness of health issues	0.218	207
Q18. Enable individuals to address issues which affect their health and well-being	0.000	209
Q19. Raise awareness of the needs of individuals discharged from your services	7.431**	207
Q20. Promote the needs of individuals in the community	10.228**	204
Q21. Negotiate, agree and support placements for individuals	8.027**	205
Q22. Develop, monitor and review discharge packages to manage individuals	14.328***	206
Q23. Contribute to the provision of effective physical, social and emotional environments for group care	1.386	206
Q24. Build and sustain relationships with individuals to reinforce their therapeutic goals	0.372	206
Q25. Physically intervene in situations where there is a breakdown in environments and relationships to limit risks to those involved	0.627	206
Q26. Support individuals with difficult or potentially difficult relationships	1.685	205
Q27. Enable individuals to maintain contacts in isolating situations	0.568	203
Q28. Enable individuals to adjust to and manage their loss	0.797	203
Q29. Enable individuals' partners, relatives and friends to adjust to and manage the individual's loss	9.844**	203
Q30. Enable individuals, their partners, relatives and friends to explore and manage change	9.141**	204
Q31. Contribute to establishing and running mutual support networks	3.164	201
Q32. Support individuals when they are distressed	0.000	206
Q33. Create and maintain boundaries between the community and individuals detained in secure conditions	13.579***	201
Q34. Protect patients from themselves and each other	1.285	205
Q35. Contribute to the protection of individuals from abuse	0.025	204
Q36. Escort patients within and beyond secure settings	1.217	205

Q37. Manage one's caseload against the prioritised needs of individuals	0.310	202
Q38. Support and lead teams to enable work objectives to be met	1.943	202
Q39. Support staff in maintaining their identity and safe personal boundaries	0.085	206
Q40. Counsel and support staff in times of stress	0.537	204
Q41. Promote, monitor and maintain health, safety and security in the workplace	0.014	208
Q42. Receive, transmit, store and retrieve information	0.000	206
Q43. Contribute to the development of knowledge and practice	0.000	208
Q44. Develop oneself within the role	0.000	208
Q45. Contribute to the development of others	0.451	208

$[\chi^2$ = **chi-square incorporating Yates' correction for continuity; * significant (<0.05); ** highly significant (<0.01); *** very highly significant (<0.001)]**

Chi-square results comparing high secure and regional secure units for level of importance reported (df=1).

Competency	χ^2	N
Q1. Promote people's equality, diversity and rights	0.066	209
Q2. Promote effective communication and relationships	0.003	210
Q3. Promote communication with individuals where there are communication differences	0.588	207
Q4. Assess individuals to determine their overall needs and risk	0.256	210
Q5. Provide specialist assessment services on individuals' needs so that others can take action	0.000	189
Q6. Assist in the assessment of, and the planning of programmes of care for, individuals	1.266	209
Q7. Plan specific therapeutic interventions to enable individuals to recognise and address any socially-unacceptable behaviour	1.215	211
Q8. Contribute to the joint implementation and monitoring of programmes of care for individuals	1.240	210
Q9. Implement specific therapeutic interventions to enable individuals to manage their behaviour	1.889	209
Q10. Assist in the implementation and monitoring of specific therapeutic interventions	1.1835	208
Q11. Enable individuals to develop and maintain skills of independent living	0.435	208
Q12. Enable individuals to develop meaningful relationships with others	1.494	199
Q13. Enable individuals who are at risk to themselves and others to identify behavioural boundaries and develop control	0.814	208
Q14. Contribute to the evaluation and improvement of programmes of care for individuals	1.197	208
Q15. Assess individuals' needs for primary health care services	0.000	187
Q16. Develop, monitor and review programmes of primary health care for individuals	0.101	182
Q17. Contribute to raising awareness of health issues	0.124	201
Q18. Enable individuals to address issues which affect their health and well-being	2.001	205
Q19. Raise awareness of the needs of individuals discharged from your services	0.024	186
Q20. Promote the needs of individuals in the community	2.462	156
Q21. Negotiate, agree and support placements for individuals	0.000	173
Q22. Develop, monitor and review discharge packages to manage individuals	0.043	172
Q23. Contribute to the provision of effective physical, social and emotional environments for group care	2.217	196
Q24. Build and sustain relationships with individuals to reinforce their therapeutic goals	3.208	206
Q25. Physically intervene in situations where there is a breakdown in environments and relationships to limit risks to those involved	1.157	205
Q26. Support individuals with difficult or potentially difficult relationships	0.813	203
Q27. Enable individuals to maintain contacts in isolating situations	1.760	197
Q28. Enable individuals to adjust to and manage their loss	0.415	193
Q29. Enable individuals' partners, relatives and friends to adjust to and manage the individual's loss	0.275	185
Q30. Enable individuals, their partners, relatives and friends to explore and manage change	0.000	182
Q31. Contribute to establishing and running mutual support networks	0.064	151
Q32. Support individuals when they are distressed	3.148	208
Q33. Create and maintain boundaries between the community and individuals detained in secure conditions	0.000	170
Q34. Protect patients from themselves and each other	3.799	204
Q35. Contribute to the protection of individuals from abuse	2.695	206
Q36. Escort patients within and beyond secure settings	3.629	200

Q37. Manage one's caseload against the prioritised needs of individuals	1.295	187
Q38. Support and lead teams to enable work objectives to be met	1.451	192
Q39. Support staff in maintaining their identity and safe personal boundaries	1.777	202
Q40. Counsel and support staff in times of stress	2.149	202
Q41. Promote, monitor and maintain health, safety and security in the workplace	3.178	207
Q42. Receive, transmit, store and retrieve information	2.748	204
Q43. Contribute to the development of knowledge and practice	3.207	209
Q44. Develop oneself within the role	4.218*	210
Q45. Contribute to the development of others	3.695	207

[χ^2 = chi-square incorporating Yates' correction for continuity; * significant (<0.05); ** highly significant (<0.01); *** very highly significant (<0.001)]

APPENDIX 5.6

Audit Results

1. Competencies required of Nurses in secure settings:

ITEM	STANDARD	AUDIT			
		Yes	No	Check	Ask
1.1	The grade mix of staff is related to the needs of the Patients.	16	2	Rotas	Staff on Duty
1.2	The experience of staff is taken into account.	18		Rotas	Staff on Duty
1.3	Staff are able to determine the difference between physical security & relational security	18			Staff on Duty
1.4	Flexible staffing systems are arranged around the needs of the patient.	14	4	Rotas	
1.5	All wards have appropriate resources to minimise/intervene in episodes of violence or dangerous behaviour.	16	2	Policy File	Staff on Duty
1.6	All staff are familiar with security policies and take personal responsibility for security issues.	18			Staff on Duty
1.7	Each registered nurse has access to their specific job description	15	3		Staff on Duty
1.8	A copy of current nursing job descriptions are available on the ward/dept for reference	8	10	Ask for copy	
1.9	The ward/dept has undergone a skill/grade mix review in the last 3 years	13	5	Ask for copy	
1.10	There are sufficient qualified nurses to meet the provision of care in line with the nursing objectives	15	3	Rotas	
1.11	The ward can claim adequate supervision of novices and students by:				
1.11.1	At least one nurse is trained in clinical supervision techniques	12	6		Nurse to be identified
1.11.2	At least one nurse is trained in Teaching and Assessing techniques	15	3		Nurse to be identified
1.11.3	At least one nurse is a trained preceptor	10	8		Nurse to be identified
1.12	Recruitment procedures are consistent with equal opportunities legislation	17	1	Policy File	
1.13	Nurses have a clear line of managerial accountability	18			Copy of Organisational Chart

2. Are Nursing Interventions Evidence Based?

ITEM	STANDARD	AUDIT			
		Yes	No	Check	Ask
2.1	A resource file of pertinent research papers to the area of clinical practice is kept on the ward	15	3	Examine File	
2.2	The resource file is varied and up to current date	13	5	Examine File	
2.3	Research papers are disseminated to ward level and are stored for reference and are easily accessible	14	4	Examine File	
2.4	Nurses have demonstrated a need for change through research	15	3	Evidence of change	
2.5	Nursing policies and procedures reflect current knowledge, research findings and principles of nursing practice with all reference sources demonstrated	15	3	Policy File	

3.   The Development of Practice Standards:

ITEM	STANDARD	AUDIT			
		Yes	No	Check	Ask
3.1	At least one member of the ward team has been instructed in Standard Setting and acts as a resource to the ward team	13	5		Nurse to be identified
3.2	Standards are audited by the ward team at least twice a year and necessary changes implemented.	9	9	Ask for copy	
3.3	Standards are reviewed every 12 months by the ward team.	12	6	Ask for copy	
3.4	Ward staff are aware of the standards of care.	18			Staff on Duty
3.5	Ward standards are displayed for patients' information.	9	9	Notice Board	
3.6	Each ward has a nursing policies and procedures file	17	1	Policy File	
3.7	Staff are satisfied with their level of involvement in the development of policies and procedures	8	10		Staff on Duty
3.8	Local policies and procedures are consistent with legislation affecting nursing practice and current professional guidelines	17	1	Policy File	
3.9	Each new patient has a written assessment carried out by a registered nurse within an agreed time-scale	17	1	Care Plan	
3.10	Each patient and family has access to a named nurse	14	4	Care Plan	Patients
3.11	Nurses receive clear written operational guidance which is regularly reviewed and includes:				
3.11.1	The nurses role, function and contribution to the assessment process, including risk assessment, care planning and discharge arrangements for patients	17	1	Policy File	Staff on Duty
3.11.2	Arrangements to meet responsibilities arising from relevant legislation and guidance	18		Policy File	Staff on Duty
3.11.3	Equal opportunities strategy	17	1	Policy File	
3.11.4	The protection of patients rights	18		Policy File	Patients
3.11.5	The nurse's contribution to treatment	18		Policy File	Staff on Duty
3.11.6	Safety and security aspects	17	1	Policy File	Staff on Duty
3.11.7	Record keeping, access to records and confidentiality	18		Policy File	Staff on Duty
3.12	Systems are in place to monitor the cost, efficiency and effectiveness of nursing in meeting its objectives and priorities	16	2	Ask for copy	Staff on Duty

4.   The Preparation given to Nurses:

ITEM	STANDARD	AUDIT			
		Yes	No	Check	Ask
4.1	All ward-based staff have undergone an induction course organised by their new employers.	14	4	Details of Course	Staff on Duty
4.2	All staff have undergone a ward-based induction.	16	2	Details of programme	Staff on Duty
4.3	Newly appointed nurses have received an information pack (reviewed every 3 years) with the following information;	14	4	Details of pack	
4.3.1	Details of post and job description	14	4	Details of pack	
4.3.2	The line of accountability	18		Details of pack	
4.3.3	The qualifications required and grade of the post	18		Details of pack	
4.3.4	The functions and responsibilities of the post (including Quality issues)	18		Details of pack	
4.3.5	The frequency of Individual performance review	18		Details of pack	
4.3.6	The terms and conditions of service	15	3	Details of pack	
4.3.7	The profile of the ward/dept initially posted to	16	2	Details of pack	
4.4	New employees receive a mandatory period of 2 weeks supernumerary induction	13	5	Details of Course	Staff on Duty
4.5	Newly employed but qualified nurses not having worked in the last 5 years attend a mandatory return to practice course	3*	1*	Details of pack	Staff on Duty
4.6	Newly qualified nurses attend and complete workshops and portfolio work for the preceptorship programme	3*	3*	Details of programme	Staff on Duty
4.7	Novices involved in preceptorship receive regular clinical supervision from the named preceptor at least fortnightly	4*	2*	Details of programme	Staff on Duty
4.8	Each nurse has a named clinical supervisor	6	12	Details of programme	Staff on Duty
4.9	Nurses take part in some form of clinical supervision at least once a month	3	15	Details of programme	Staff on Duty
4.9.1	Nurses take part in some form of clinical supervision at least once every 3 months on request	11	7	Details of programme	Staff on Duty
4.10	The ward induction booklet/profile contains evidence supporting:				
4.10.1	The profile of the ward/dept	17	1	Induction Material	Staff on Duty

4.10.2	The nursing philosophy	18		Induction Material	Staff on Duty
4.10.3	Induction materials and checklists	15	3	Induction Material	Staff on Duty
4.11	There exists a staff development programme which includes requirements for continuing training, links with forensic and other nursing outside the unit and other opportunities for professional growth	16	2	Details of programme	Staff on Duty
4.12	The training programme includes:				
4.12.1	Issues in relation to gender, sexual orientation, race and culture, religion, language, age and ability	15	3	Details of programme	
4.12.2	The assessment of risk and dangerousness	17	1	Details of programme	
4.12.3	Safe practice guidelines	18		Details of programme	
4.12.4	Mental health legislation and guidance	14	4	Details of programme	
4.12.5	The drawing up of an annual training programme for each nurse	14	4	Details of programme	Staff on Duty
4.12.6	Care and responsibility	15	3	Details of programme	
4.12.7	De-escalation techniques	13	5	Details of programme	

* Many of the organisations had not employed newly qualified or returners to practice.

5. Working with difficult patients

ITEM	STANDARD	AUDIT			
		Yes	No	Check	Ask
5.1	Staff integrate with patients whilst being aware of security needs.	18			Staff on Duty
5.2	There is a policy on the handling of violent incidents.	16	2	Policy File	
5.3	Staff are aware of the policy for handling violent incidents	16	2		Staff on Duty
5.4	Members of the ward team have attended a Control & Restraint course	15	3		Staff on Duty
5.5	Nurses have knowledge of the patients within the ward and are able to minimise patients disturbed behaviour.	18			Staff on Duty
5.6	The ward has an identified seclusion procedure	13	5*	Policy File	
5.7	Nurses are aware of the seclusion policy.	14	4*		Staff on Duty
5.8	There is a post-incident discussion with the patient.	13	5*		Staff on Duty
5.9	The rights of detained patients are ensured under the provision of the 1983 Mental Health Act	12	6*		Patients
5.10	Individual safety and security needs are reviewed to meet the changing needs of the patient	18		Care Plan	Staff on Duty
5.11	Individual safety and security needs are clearly written within the treatment plan	17	1	Care Plan	
5.12	The ward has an identified procedure for Special Observation	14	4*	Policy File	
5.13	Staff de-briefing is available following a serious incident	18			Staff on Duty
5.14	Members of the ward team have received instruction on use of de-escalation techniques	13	5		Staff on Duty

* Some Health Care Centres within the Prison Services do not have in-patients, therefore seclusion and observation procedures are not appropriate.

6. Utilising UKCC Policies to inform practice:

ITEM	STANDARD	AUDIT			
		Yes	No	Check	Ask
6.1	Copies of all leading UKCC and Professional documents are held on the ward for easy reference			Policy File	
6.2	Code of Professional Conduct	16	2	Policy File	
6.3	Guidelines for Record Keeping	7	11	Policy File	
6.4	Guidelines regarding Accountability	11	7	Policy File	
6.5	Scope of Professional Practice	13	5	Policy File	
6.6	Guidelines for mental Health and Learning Disability Nursing	11	7	Policy File	
6.7	PREP guidelines	11	7	Policy File	
6.8	Making a Complaint	13	5	Policy File	
6.9	Guidelines regarding Confidentiality	7	11	Policy File	
6.10	Standards for Administering Medicines	13	5	Policy File	
6.10.1	There is a procedure for safe custody, prescribing and administration of drugs.	17	1	Policy File	
6.10.2	Drug keys are kept in the appropriate secure place	18			Person in Charge
6.10.3	Staff are aware of the safe keeping of drugs	18			Staff on Duty
6.10.4	Drugs are stored in accordance with the medicine procedures	17	1	Drug Storage	
6.10.5	A record of errors is kept and is available for reference	4	14	Records	
6.10.6	The record of errors book demonstrates the investigation of the cause of error and the outcome, identifying actions taken to avoid re-occurrence	4	14	Records	
6.10.7	Prescriptions are clearly written, typed or computer generated and entries are indelible and dated	14	4	Prescription Sheets	
6.10.8	Where a new prescription replaces earlier prescriptions the latter have been cancelled clearly and the cancellation signed and dated by an authorised medical practitioner	13	5	Prescription Sheets	
6.10.9	The prescription provides clear and unequivocal identification of the patient for whom the medicine is intended	16	2	Prescription Sheets	
6.10.10	There is a clear procedure for identification of the patient	13	5	Policy File	Staff on Duty
6.10.11	The substance to be administered is clearly specified	18		Prescription Sheets	

6.10.12	The form has been clearly stated (e.g. tablet, syrup etc.)	17	1	Prescription Sheets	
6.10.13	The administration of unprescribed medicines is covered by a recognised protocol agreed between managers, nurses, pharmacists and medical practitioners	16	2	Policy File	
6.11	The nurse in charge of the ward/unit is able to satisfy themselves that all registered nurses in their charge are				
6.11.1	Knowledgeable and understanding of the substances used for therapeutic purposes	18			Staff on Duty
6.11.2	Able to justify any actions they take	18			Staff on Duty
6.11.3	Prepared to be accountable for any actions they take	18			Staff on Duty
6.11.4	Knowledgeable regarding the identity of patients	18			Person in Charge
6.11.5	Aware of the patients current assessment and planned programme of care	17	1		Person in Charge
6.11.6	Pay due regard to the environment in which care is given	18			Staff on Duty
6.11.7	Carefully scrutinise the written prescription and the information provided on relevant containers	18			Staff on Duty
6.11.8	Able to question and challenge the medical practitioner or pharmacist if the prescription or container is illegible, unclear, ambiguous or incomplete or falls outside the product licence and where believed necessary to refuse to administer a prescribed substance	18		Policy File	Staff on Duty
6.11.9	Refuse to prepare substances for injection in advance of their immediate use	18		Policy File	Staff on Duty
6.11.10	Refuse to administer a medicine not placed in a container or drawn into a syringe by them or in their presence	18			Staff on Duty
6.12	The ward displays a range of patient information leaflets concerning their prescribed medicines	2	16	Display	
6.13	The nurse in charge of the ward is able to satisfy themselves of the competency of each registered nurse to:				
6.13.1	Check the expiry date of any medicine	18		Monitoring	Person in Charge
6.13.2	Carefully consider the dosage, method of administration, route and timing of administration in the context of the specific patient at the operative time	17	1	Monitoring	Person in Charge

6.13.3	Carefully consider whether any of the prescribed medicines may dangerously interact with each other	18		Monitoring	Person in Charge
6.13.4	Determine whether it is necessary to withhold a medicine pending consultation with the prescribing medical practitioner	18		Monitoring	Person in Charge
6.13.5	Contact the prescriber without delay where the contra-indications of the medicine are observed	18		Monitoring	Person in Charge
6.13.6	Make clear and accurate records of the administration of all medicines administered or deliberately withheld	18		Records	Person in Charge
6.13.7	Where a medicine is refused by a patient assess the consequences and inform the prescriber accordingly	17	1	Records	
6.13.8	Use the opportunity which administration of medicine provides for emphasising to patients and carers the importance and implications of the prescribed treatment and for enhancing their understanding of its effects and side effects	16	2		Staff on Duty
6.13.9	Make accurate records of the positive and negative effects of the medicine, making these known to the prescribing medical practitioner	16	2	Records	
6.13.10	Honestly acknowledge personal limitations and seek further advice whenever this is felt to be necessary	17	1	Records	Staff on Duty

7. Practice issues relevant to physical health needs

ITEM	STANDARD	AUDIT			
		Yes	No	Check	Ask
7.1	Interpretation services are available if required.	12	4		Staff/ Patients
7.2	Nurses are aware of patients with hearing loss and can respond to communication.	17	1	Care Plan	
7.3	Nurses are aware of patients who have difficulties with verbal communication and can respond accordingly	17	1	Care Plan	
7.4	All patients receive nursing care and treatment that is designed to meet each individuals needs in an appropriate and non-discriminatory manner.	17	1	Care Plan	
7.5	Records indicate that additional support is provided where appropriate e.g. chiropodist, Dietician, Optician, Speech Therapist	17	1	Care Plan	
7.6	Specific advice and/or clinics are provided on issues such as asthma and diabetes	15	3		Staff/ Patients
7.7	Patients are given the opportunity to access fresh air and exercise	18		Policy File	Patients
7.8	There is an identified Health Promotion nurse	12	6	Identify nurse	
7.9	Patients are offered a monthly health check at ward level (including blood pressure, urine analysis, pulse and weight) any problems highlighted are referred to the G.P	5	13	Records	Staff/ Patients
7.10	Patients are offered an annual dental check up	12	6	Records	Staff/ Patients
7.11	In the event of physical ill-health, patients have access to a G.P	14	3	Records	Staff/ Patients
7.12	Where necessary patients are transferred to a local acute NHS Trust for more specialised treatment	18		Records	Staff/ Patients
7.13	Patients have the right to request a second opinion about any aspect of their physical treatment	16	2	Policy File	Staff/ Patients
7.14	Patients who require a particular type of diet to suit their religious/cultural/dietary needs are provided with them	16	2	Care Plan	Patients
7.15	Patients can expect information to be in plain language and, where necessary, in languages other than English and in forms which people with sight, hearing , learning or other disabilities can use	16	1	Policy File	Staff/ Patients
7.16	If patients have problems with hearing or speech, or their first language is not English, they can expect help in getting access to services, including where appropriate, interpreting services	18		Policy File	Staff/ Patients
7.17	People have a choice in being treated by a health professional of their own gender	17	1	Policy File	Staff/ Patients
7.18	The patients preferences are documented in the care plan and the individuals spiritual and cultural needs are taken into consideration with details noted	17	1	Care Plan	Staff/ Patients
7.19	Nurses demonstrate awareness of, and sensitivity to the issues associated with gender, sexual orientation, race and culture, religion, language, age and ability	18			Staff/ Patients

Report to the
UKCC Commission
for Education

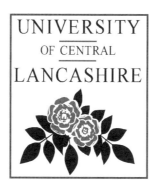

University of Central Lancashire
Faculty of Health

Nursing in Secure Environments Project

Report to UKCC Commission

Synopsis

1   This paper presents preliminary findings from a series of research activities aimed at reviewing the effectiveness of the preparation currently given to nurses working in secure environments. The paper presents findings from focus groups, focus interviews and a survey questionnaire. Key themes from this are identified. For further information on this paper contact Richard Bradshaw, Professional Officer, Mental Health and Learning Disabilities Nursing on 0171 333 6546.

Recommended action

2   The committee is invited to:

2.1   receive this paper for information; and

2.2   discuss the most appropriate way for this information to be presented to the UKCC's Education Commission.

Background

3   The Nursing in Secure Environments Project was commissioned by the UKCC in April 1998, commenced in July 1998 and reports to Council in June 1999.

4   The project will assist in Council's endeavours by helping to clarify accountability for the Registered Nurse practitioner in secure settings. These are services where there is a need to balance the needs of a patient or client for health and social care, with the security expectations of society.

5   The project reflects the fact that there is an emerging need for staff skills to be made generalisable and transferable to a variety of secure settings including the public,

private and voluntary sectors of health and social care and the criminal justice systems within the United Kingdom.

6   Key issues being addressed by the project team include:

- Describe the competencies required of nurses working in secure environments

- How effective is the preparation currently given to nurses working in secure environments

7   The objective of the scoping exercise is to provide a comprehensive overview of the educational, occupational and professional practice expectations placed on nurses working in secure environments. This would include both secure health and Prison Services at all levels of security across the UK.

Methodologies Used

Literature search

8   An exploratory review of the literature relating to forensic care and the use and development of standards was conducted. This encompassed the main electronic sources of medical, nursing and social sciences literature. In addition, hand searching and examination of unpublished 'grey literature', together with Internet searches, was carried out to enhance the validity of the literature review.

Focus groups

9   Focus groups are a form of group interview that capitalise on communication between research participants in order to generate data. This explicitly uses group interaction as part of the method and people are encouraged to talk to one another: asking questions, exchanging anecdotes and commenting on each other's experiences and points of view.

10   Most focus group studies use a theoretical sampling model whereby participants are selected to reflect a range of the total study population or to test particular hypotheses and this was the approach adopted. At analysis this method draws together and compares discussions of similar themes and examines how these relate to the variables within the sample population. (A list of organisations represented at the focus groups is at Annexe 1 and 2)

Focused interviews

11   A series of interviews were held, focused on a specific purposive sample of interviewees which can be defined as "a type of a non- probability sampling method in which the researcher selects subjects for the study on the basis of personal judgement about which ones will be most representative or productive." (Polit and Hungler 1993)

12   This interview technique was used to ensure that all subject areas are covered, and also

allows the respondents freedom of reply and description to illustrate concepts. The use of focused interviews allowed the project co-ordinators to obtain detailed personal reactions and opinions. (A list of interviews undertaken to date is at Annexe 3)

<u>Questionnaires</u>

13   Questionnaires have been distributed to sixty five education providers across the United Kingdom. The questionnaires were sent to programme leaders for Mental Health and learning Disabilities programmes, in the questionnaires we sought information about theory and practice content in relation to Mentally Disordered Offenders within pre-registration and post- registration programmes. An analysis of the responses to date has been prepared which is included later in this paper.

Defining Secure Environments

14   In undertaking this project the criteria that defined "secure environments" both within the health and criminal justice sectors needed clarification. The definitions and criteria outlined by the Mental Health Foundation (1998) in their series of guides *Commissioning Services for Offenders with Mental Health Problems* provided us with a base from which to work within the Health Sector.

15   Secure environments are provided both within the public and private sectors of health care and the Prison Services. The criteria for admission or detention in these facilities are described below:

<u>Health</u>

15.1   Within the health sector secure environments are provided for patients who have mental health problems or learning disabilities. Secure environments are provided at low, medium and high levels within the appropriate mental health legislation for England and Wales (Mental Health Act 1983), The Mental Health (Scotland) Act 1984 and The Mental Health (Northern Ireland) Act 1986. The legislation is fundamentally parallel across the four countries, the key aspects which impact on the project is the way that personality disordered offenders are recognised within the legislation.

<u>Criminal Justice</u>

15.2   In the Prison Services in England and Wales there are 157 establishments, Scotland has 19 establishments and Northern Ireland 4. The level of health care provided varies but can be generalised as:

- Health Care Centre   1   9 am-5 p.m. (approx.) primary care and out patient facilities

- Health Care Centre   2   7 am-9 p.m. (approx.) primary care and out patient facilities

- Health Care Centre   3   24 hours in patient facilities

15.3   In addressing the issues of competencies needed and the effectiveness of educational preparation for working in secure environments it is necessary to identify the uniqueness of the work of nurses in prison settings.

15.4   A prime difference between nurses working in prisons and nurses working in any other arena is that nurses working in prison do not have total control over the types of patient that they are nursing.

15.5   In a medical ward in an acute hospital a nurse knows that a patient will generally present with a medical condition, can be nursed by a nurse who has developed skills knowledge and understanding of medical nursing developed through an educational programme that has been designed to address these needs.

15.6   Whereas in prison settings a nurse may be presented with patients who have a medical condition, have a mental illness or personality disorder. Tomorrow the patients will be different and the nursing problems they present are different. A prison nurse needs to be able to assess, plan, implement and evaluate care for patients who in other settings would be nursed by nurses who are on different parts of the UKCC Register.

Findings from Focus Groups and Focused Interviews and Literature Search

16   During the initial data capture we have met with over 250 nurses from secure environments at all levels across the four UK countries. From the Focus Groups and focused interviews there is a general feeling that current pre-registration programmes not only fail to prepare people for working in secure environments, but also they do not adequately prepare nurses, at the point of initial registration, with the skills required in the workplace.

17   It would be inappropriate to identify individuals who have made the following comments as they were assured of confidentiality in a bid to encourage openness and honesty from the participants. Comments made include:

> "Project 2000 seems to be preparing managers"

> "They have intellectualised nursing"

> "Most students get their knowledge about forensic psychiatry through the newspapers, the same as the general public"

> "There are nurses qualifying who do not know their basic drugs, for example they have never given depots"

> "Tutorial staff are discouraging students from undertaking placements in secure settings"

> "Students are of extremes, some excellent some very poor"

> "Tutors have insufficient knowledge to guide students"

"We are not preparing people for working in this area, but should we be, there is a view that current pre-reg programmes do not prepare people for working in general mental health areas. I would like to see more emphasis on Forensic issues in pre-reg"

"One cannot expect basic nurse training to go to sufficient depth to cover offending behaviour and the way services are provided, and the link between agencies in criminal justice and health"

"Project 2000 has helped nurses express themselves better"

"We need to look closely at our expectations of outcomes of the diploma programme"

"We should not expect students to come out of a pre-registration programme and take responsibility for a ward"

"CFP should be one year and then allow more time for specialist mental health issues, with possibly 3 months in a range of placements with Mentally Disordered Offenders"

"Pre-reg is focused on community care. When people qualify they have very little knowledge and experience of institutional care and the needs of patients in institutions"

"Education providers don't know what we need"

"I don't think they are prepared to work in any environment"

18   Many of these views are supported in the literature, May et al 1997 report that there is an over emphasis on theory within the programmes and that theory and practice are not linked. This coupled with the number of short placements available to students reduces their ability to develop the appropriate skills.

19   The ENB guidance to education providers, *Creating Lifelong Learners- Partnership for Care (1994)* highlights the need for students "to develop their skills and to gain the necessary confidence, they need to have experience of caring for people with a variety of mental illnesses across the age range. Examples include mentally disordered offenders, people who abuse substances...people with challenging behaviour" (ENB 1994). However from an early analysis of our research data, extracted from questionnaires completed by education providers, we have found a significant variance in this criteria being applied. Some education institutions provide an opportunity for students to undertake a 13 week elective in a secure environment, others include a shorter placement as an integral part of the mental health or learning disabilities branch whilst some institutions only provide a single lecture on the issue of Mentally Disordered Offenders.

20   When asked what should be a minimum requirement for inclusion in pre-registration programmes, participants in the focus groups and focused interviews, varied greatly in the range of input to the programme. This range included the view at one extreme, that there should be a Forensic Mental Health Branch through to lectures from practitioners at the other extreme.

21   The literature search also highlighted a number of points, the Reed Report
      (Department of Health 1994) made a number of recommendations including:

      •   that training courses for community psychiatric nurses include consideration
           of forensic nursing issues and opportunities for placement in forensic settings

      •   that the ENB considers the future need for Project 2000 training in forensic
           psychiatric nursing, including opportunities for suitable placements

      •   that prisons continue to forge closer links with local hospitals, colleges of
           nursing and others who can assist in the development of nurse education.

22   Reed (1994) also predicted that "it is likely that they (Project 2000 students) will have
      received rather less specialised training than their RMN and RMNH predecessors,
      while opportunities for practical experience of the range of problems found among
      psychiatric in-patients are increasingly limited due to the provision of services away
      from hospitals. It is reasonable to assume, therefore, that Project 2000 students would
      require some additional education in forensic psychiatric issues, although greater
      emphasis should now be given to such opportunities as part of post-registration
      training".

23   Mentally Disordered Offenders are in contact with a wide range of mental health
      services from community programmes and diversion schemes through to in-patient
      facilities in high secure hospitals. With this in mind we feel that there should be
      consideration given to increasing the knowledge and skills base in relation to MDOs
      within the Mental Health and Learning Disabilities Branch programmes.

24   During the course of the project we have had discussion with over 250 nurses,
      working in secure settings within the health care and criminal justice sectors, and a
      general belief is held that pre-registration fails to meet the needs of the service, the
      Common Foundation programme is too long and too adult focused and students
      frequently lack the practical, communication and inter-personal skills required for
      practice. Again these views are supported within the literature, et al (1995), May et al
      (1997) recommended that there was an increase in mental health and learning
      disability content within CFP and that counselling skills and stress management
      would benefit all students. The authors Eraut et al (1995), May et al (1997) McEvoy
      (1995) and the Sainsbury Centre for Mental Health (1997) also suggest that the length
      of the CFP should be altered to either a one year or a six month period.

The Education Providers Questionnaire

Introduction

25   One of the key themes of the UKCC Nursing in Secure Environments project centred
      on the educational preparation of nurses to work in these settings ("How effective is
      the preparation currently given to nurses working in secure environments?" UKCC
      1998). In considering this item a key area of educational preparation was identified at
      pre-registration. It was clear from the literature search that no previous study had
      examined this issue and that to gain a current picture of pre-registration preparation
      empirical research needed to be conducted.

26   A questionnaire was designed and piloted in the north-west of England at the University of Central Lancashire. A number of subject specialists were also contacted and provided commentary and feedback. The final questionnaire, approved by the project and steering committees of the project, was circulated to institutions offering pre-registration preparation for the Mental Health and Learning Disabilities branch programmes throughout the UK from information provided by the four National Boards. In all 27 responses have been received to date, which constituted 41.5 per cent of the total sample. This response falls well within the expected return for a study of this nature and would be regarded as an adequate sample on which to draw conclusions.

The Respondents

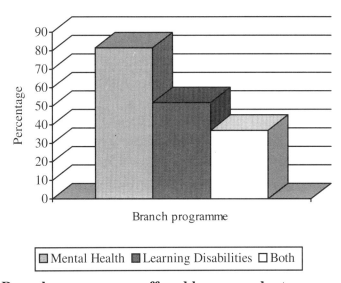

Figure 1: Branch programmes offered by respondents

27   Of the 27 respondents 23 responses were received from English education providers, 3 from Scotland, 1 from Northern Ireland and none from Wales.

28   In all 22 of the respondents were offering the Mental Health Branch programme, 14 the Learning Disability Branch programme with 10 respondents offering both Branches (see figure 1).

Practice Placements

29   Respondents were asked a number of key questions in relation to the placement of pre-registration students for clinical practice in secure environments. In all 81% of the respondents offered placements in secure environments, with 19% not offering this opportunity (see figure 2). The placements ranged from three to sixteen weeks in length with a mean of 7.65 weeks.

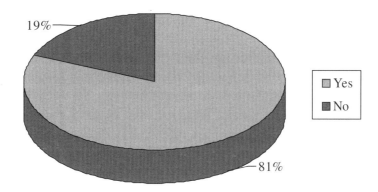

Figure 2: Respondents offering placement in secure setting

30   In response to the question concerning the type of placements, 10 different types of facility were identified. Six of these facilities were included in the original questionnaire with an opportunity for respondents to add others not listed.

31   The most common placement for students was in a Medium Secure Unit, with eighteen respondents utilising these placements. This was followed by intensive care units (nine respondents) and high dependency units (eight respondents). A number of prisons had been utilised for placements (six respondents) and a small number of respondents had placements in the high security Special Hospitals (six respondents). These latter figures may reflect the location of the educational establishments with those near to the Special Hospitals likely to make use of these facilities. The additional facilities identified by respondents included: a low secure unit; forensic services, admission/assessment unit, clinical therapies department. These additional facilities were only identified by single respondents and again may reflect the current development of services within a given locality. With the current development of forensic services nationally it is likely that this configuration of placements could change considerably over the next three to five years. The expansion of community forensic services, low security units, increased medium secure unit beds, intensive care facilities and twenty four hour nursed beds becoming available (Dept of Health 1998) will mean increased opportunity and scope for local practice placements.

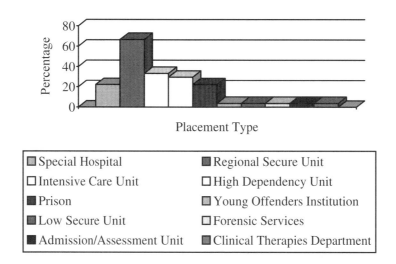

Figure 3: Type of Practice Placement

32   Further analysis of the placement use identified that the majority of the respondents are using more than one type of secure environment for clinical placements. Nearly 60 per cent of respondents were using more than one facility with the most common usage being two (25.9%) and 3 (22.2%) see Table 1. This again may reflect the disparity of forensic service development and clinical experience in secure environment is not as limited to larger institutions as it once was.

Number of placements used	N	%
None	5	18.5
One	6	22.2
Two	7	25.9
Three	6	22.2
Four	2	7.4
Five	0	0.0
Six	1	3.7
Total	**27**	**100.0**

Table 1: Number of Placements used by Respondents

33   Respondents were asked at what stage of the students training they undertook a placement in a secure environment. As expected the majority of the placements were in the latter part of the course, i.e. the third year with twenty respondents (74 per cent) reporting placement at that stage of training (see Figure 4). A high number of placement however did take place during the second your of training (twelve respondents) and a small number in the first year (two respondents). Given the current structure of pre-registration education this reflects more frequent placements during the last 18 months of the branch programmes rather than the earlier stages of the Common Foundation Programme.

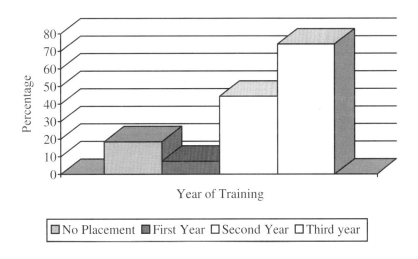

Figure 4: Stage of Training Students undertake Secure placement

34   When the data was further analysed to examine whether placements were taking place in more than one year it was noted that the majority (twelve respondents) use placement in one year only (see table 2). Eight respondents however (56.4 per cent) were offering placements during a combination of the second and third years. A small minority of respondents (two, equalling 9%) offered placements in a combination of the first and second, first and third and in one case placements in all years of training.

Years that placements are offered	N	% of those which offer
One year only	12	54.5
First and second years	2	9.0
First and third years	2	9.0
Second and third years	8	36.4
All years	2	9.0

Table 2: Stage of Training for Placement in a Secure Environment

35   Education providers were asked whether a placement in a secure environment was an optional or integral part of the pre-registration programme. The majority of respondents offer these placements on an optional basis to students (twelve respondents equalling 44 per cent) with eight respondents (equalling 29%) offering them as an integral part of the program (see Table 3). A small number of respondents (three equalling 11%) offered this as both an integral and optional part of the programme (it is presumed that there is a mandatory part of the programme with an option for the student at a later stage in the training to take a further placement).

Placement	N	%
Neither	4	14.8
Optional	12	44.4
Integral	8	29.6
Both	3	11.1
Total	27	100.0

Table 3: Are Placements Optional or Integral?

The Educational Environment

36   Education providers were asked whether they had set learning outcomes in relation to theory and practice for nursing people in secure settings. The analysis of responses showed that ten (37 per cent) had neither objectives for theory nor practice. One respondent stated that they had outcomes for practice alone and a further six respondents (22 per cent) have learning outcomes for theory alone. Only ten of the respondents (37 per cent) had learning outcomes for both theory and practice for nursing people in secure settings (see Table 4).

37   In addition education providers were asked to estimate what percentage of their programme was devoted to theory and practice for nursing people in secure settings. The majority (fourteen respondents equalling 52%) either did not provide an estimate or in a few cases (four) stated they could not estimate this. The respondents to this question showed a range from one to fifteen per cent with a mean of 5.08%.

Learning Outcomes for Theory and Practice	N	% of those which offer
Neither	10	37.0
Practice	1	3.7
Theory	6	22.2
Theory and Practice	10	37.0
Total	27	100.0

Table 4: Learning Outcomes in Theory and Practice for Secure Environments

38   The education providers were asked similar questions in relation to learning outcomes in theory and practice for nursing mental disorder offenders. The figures are very similar to those given for nursing people in secure settings with slight variation (see Table 5). Eleven respondents said that they had neither learning outcomes for theory nor practice (40 per cent). One respondent said that they had learning outcomes for practice alone and a further seven respondents said they had outcomes for theory alone (26 per cent). Only eight respondents said they had learning outcomes for both theory and practice in relation to mentally disordered offenders.

39   Education providers were also asked to estimate what percentage of their programme was devoted to theory and practice for nursing mentally disordered offenders. The majority (fourteen respondents, 52%) either did not provide an estimate or in a few cases (four) stated they could not estimate this. The respondents to this question showed a range from one to fifteen per cent with a mean of 4.38%.

Learning Outcomes for Theory and Practice	N	% of those which offer
Neither	11	40.7
Practice	1	3.7
Theory	7	25.9
Theory and Practice	8	29.6
Total	27	100.0

Table 5: Learning Outcomes in Theory and Practice for Mentally Disordered Offenders

40   The results of these two questions, in relation to learning outcomes, do present major concerns in relation to the clinical placements of pre-registration students in secure environments as it would appear that a number of placements are taking place without established learning outcomes. These are only available for both theory and practice in a minority of instances (i.e. 37 per cent and 30 per cent respectively).

41   There is also a concern the wide variance and poor response in relation to the percentage of the programme devoted to both nursing in secure environments and care of mentally disordered offenders. It is clear that some pre-registration programmes are placing a much higher emphasis on this whilst others appear to be ignoring both issues completely.

The Tutorial Staff

42   The education providers were asked how many of their lecturers had clinical experience of working in a secure environment.

43   A large number of providers had no lecturers with this background (thirteen respondents, 48 per cent). Fourteen respondents had lecturing staff with such a clinical background which ranged from one lecturer in six cases: two lecturers in five cases, three lecturers in two cases and five lecturers in one case (see Figure 5).

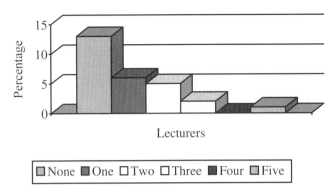

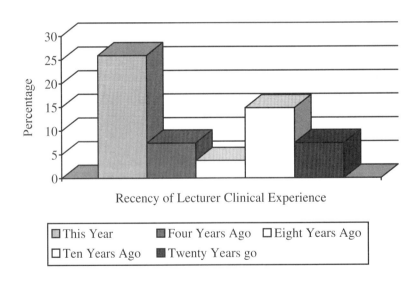

Figure 5: Number of Lecturers with Clinical experience of Secure Environments

44   A further question was asked of respondents in relation to the recency of the clinical experience of those tutorial staff with a background in secure environments. The majority of the respondents reported that their lecturers had current or recent experience of these clinical environments (seven respondents equivalent to 26 per cent). The remaining tutorial staff had experience ranging between four and twenty years ago . In detail two respondents reported experience of four years ago; one respondent experience eight years ago, four respondents with experience 10 years ago and two respondents with experience 20 years ago (see Figure 6).

Figure 6: Recency of Clinical Experience of Tutorial Staff

45   A supplementary question invited respondents to provide details of any joint appointments that they had in place. Four respondents reported a joint appointment with the majority having no such posts in place (see Figure 7).

Figure 7: Joint Educational and Service Appointments with Forensic Services

193

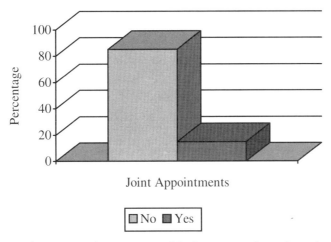

Joint Appointments

No ■ Yes

46   There appears to be a growing partnership between the education providers and local services on meeting educational need. Seven respondents, 26 per cent, reported that education programmes have input from staff employed in the local secure unit clinical services (see Figure 8). It may be useful to consider whether some of these arrangements could be formalised either by joint appointments or some other arrangement which might help both the quality and relevance of education programmes but also with the recruitment and retention of key staff.

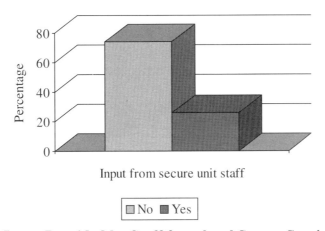

Input from secure unit staff

No ■ Yes

Figure 8: Input Provided by Staff from local Secure Services

Research Activity

47   Very few of the educational providers reported any current research programmes underway into nursing in secure environments. Four respondents in total reported positively on this item representing 15% of all respondents (see Figure 9).

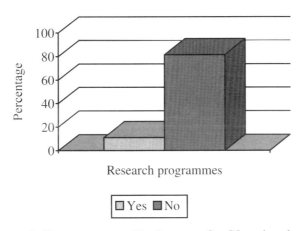

Research programmes

Yes ■ No

Figure 9: Research Programmes Underway for Nursing in Secure Environments

48   The topics covered by the research programmes reflected some of the current interest in the field of personality disorder (with two respondents reporting research in this area) and the continuing challenging area of working with women detained in secure settings. The final area of research covered multi-disciplinary working (see Table 6).

Title of Research Programme	N
Treatability of Personality Disorder	2
Education and Training needs of Staff Working with Women patients	1
Multidisciplinary Working	1

Table 6: Topics covered by Research Programmes

49   This is undoubtedly a disappointing return given that all respondents were from the Higher Education sector. This may provide a fruitful area of closer co-operation between service and educational providers for mutually supportive research and education programmes which could feed both into the practical and theoretical setting. It is difficult to see how a body of knowledge for nursing within these settings can emerge without a clear strategic approach in relation to the critical area of research.

Potential Ways Forward

50   Education providers were asked for their views on how the branch programmes might better prepare students for working in secure environment. In all twelve separate suggestions were made although in five of these instances, only a single respondent came forward with the suggestion (see Figure 10).

51   Fourteen respondents (52 per cent) expressed concerns about the time available in the branch programmes to fulfil the competing demands of the curriculum. Many stated that they had difficulties in meeting other speciality placements and that the only way that experience in secure environments or in relation to work with mental disorder offenders could be achieved was if more time was made available for the branch programme. This may be why many of the respondents suggested in response to an earlier question that experience in relation to secure environments should be optional rather than integral to the branch programme. It appears that one way educational providers cover a wider variety of experiences is via the provision of these optional routes.

52   Other key areas identified by respondents were in relation to the use of clinical placement and visits which was suggested by eight respondents equalling 30 per cent. This was suggested by respondents who already made some use of these facilities and had experienced the value of them in their branch programmes. The availability of an integrated model which had input of both theory and practice was suggested by seven respondents (25 per cent of the returns). It is already been suggested that is of major concern that some placements are taking place in the absence of structured theory and practice element.

53   Six respondents suggested the use of practitioners as lecturers which has previously been commented on as a growing trend in the branch programmes and as confirmed here as a valued way for better preparing learners for these environment. If this idea is seen as a productive way of developing this topic area in the branch programme then clear planning between service providers and education providers should take place to

ensure that this was not a token placement of a clinician in the classroom. It will be important that people are adequately prepared for this role in each environment and would therefore be able to both articulate and support learners in the most productive way.

54   These were a few specific areas identified by a small number respondents in relation to specific skills and knowledge. Three respondents identified legal and ethical issues as a way to better prepare learners (11 per cent of respondents); three respondents felt that if specific competencies could be specified these would be available for the programmes to adopt and implement, a further two respondents identified physical intervention skills as a way of better preparation.

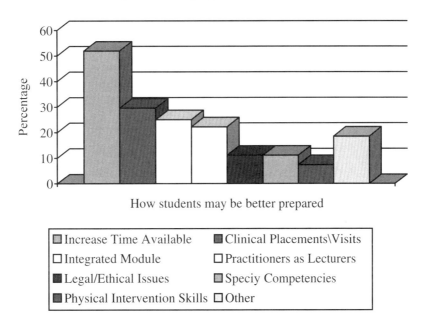

How students may be better prepared

▨ Increase Time Available	■ Clinical Placements\Visits
□ Integrated Module	□ Practitioners as Lecturers
■ Legal/Ethical Issues	▨ Speciy Competencies
■ Physical Intervention Skills	□ Other

Figure 10: How Students may be better prepared

55   The five areas identified by a single respondent included: the management of personality disorder; the empathetic use of self, the examination of applied research in this area, the attendance at conferences on this topic area, and the use of joint appointments (see Table 7).

Suggestions for Better Preparation	N	% of those which offer
Increase Time Available	14	51.9
Clinical Placements/Visits	8	29.6
Integrated Module	7	25.0
Practitioners as Lecturers	6	22.2
Legal/Ethical issues	3	11.1
Specify Competencies	3	11.1
Physical Intervention Skills	2	7.4
Managing Personality Disorder	1	3.7
Empathetic Use of Self	1	3.7
Examine Applied Research	1	3.7
Conference Attendance	1	3.7
Joint Appointment	1	3.7

Table 7: Suggestions for the better preparation of Students to work in Secure Environments

56   Education providers were asked whether they felt that the preparation for working in secure environments should be undertaken during a pre- registration programme. Fifteen of the respondents (55 per cent) stated that this preparation should take place during pre-registration whilst nine respondents (33 per cent) felt that it should not. Three respondents (equalling 11 per cent) felt unable to express a view on this matter.

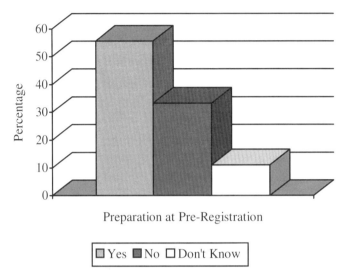

Preparation at Pre-Registration

☐ Yes ■ No ☐ Don't Know

Figure 11 : Whether preparation for working in Secure Environments should be at Pre-registration

57   The providers were asked a supplementary question in relation to this and invited to give their reasons in support of their response. In all twelve a separate reasons were given in support of why preparation should be at pre-registration and four separate reasons why they felt it should not be at pre-registration.

58   In relation to the reasons stated in support of preparation being at pre-registration five key areas were identified with a further seven mentioned by a single respondent (see Table 8). The most frequently stated reason given (eight respondents equalling 30 per cent) was that this helped to broaden the students perspective in relation to the field of mental health care and exposed them to the full spectrum of service availability. Seven respondents (26 per cent) stated that mainstream services were increasingly dealing with people with similar problems to those found in secure services and therefore it was an important experience for people on pre- registration programmes to be exposed to. Six respondents (22 per cent) mentioned that it helped students future career prospects and a number of them following the experience elected to work in secure settings. Even those choosing not to work in these settings found that it was favourably looked upon as valued experience by future employers in non- secure environments. Four respondents (15 per cent) stated that experience in secure environments provided a realistic representation of services and that it was important for students to be exposed to all aspects of care with the possibility that students could have skewed experiences by placements in community settings alone. Three respondents (11 per cent) stated that placements in a secure environment provided an opportunity to consider more rigorous risk assessment which is an increasing requirement in all mental health and learning disability services and was probably more fully developed in services dealing with high levels of mentally disordered offenders.

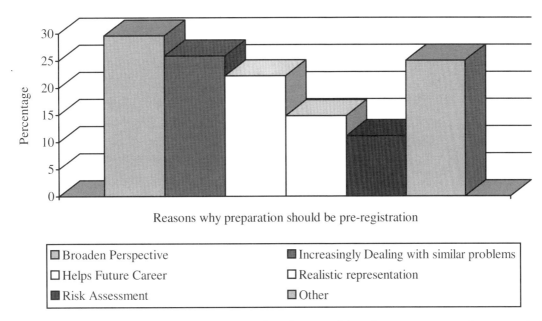

Reasons why preparation should be pre-registration

☐ Broaden Perspective	■ Increasingly Dealing with similar problems
☐ Helps Future Career	☐ Realistic representation
■ Risk Assessment	☐ Other

Figure 12: Reasons why preparation for working in a secure environment should be at pre-registration

Reasons why preparation for working in secure environments should be at pre-registration	N	% of those which offer
To Broaden Students perspective	8	29.6
Students increasingly exposed to patients with multiple problems	7	25.9
Helps with future career prospects	6	22.2
Realistic representation of services	4	14.8
Risk Assessment Opportunities	3	11.1
Good Supervision	1	3.7
Students asking for placement	1	3.7
To Develop Proactive Attitudes	1	3.7
Raise Awareness of Politics of MDO's	1	3.7
Special Needs of Carers	1	3.7
Observation Skills	1	3.7
Teamwork	1	3.7

Table 8: Reasons why preparation for working in secure environments should be at pre-registration.

59   Seven respondents came up with separate individual reasons in support of preparation at pre-registration which included: the availability of good supervision because of high staff/patient ratios and richer skill mix in secure environments; students asking for placements in these settings, to help develop good attitudes towards this difficult client group, to raise awareness of the political dimension of mentally disordered offenders, to understand the special needs of carers in relation to this complex group, the exposure to structured observation skills, and the availability of good teamwork in these environments.

60 In relation to those respondents giving reasons why preparation for working in secure environments should not be at pre- registration four areas were identified (see Figure 13). Two areas were identified by seven respondents each (equalling 26%). The first of these stated that this was a specialised area of knowledge and skills which was beyond basic education and therefore should be at post registration. The second main area was in relation to the time constraints of the curriculum stating that they felt that this topic could not be done justice ii pre-registration. This links strongly to responses to previous questions in relation to constraint on time. Two respondents commented on the limited opportunities for placements in secure environments and may reflect some local difficulties on availability. However, given the likely future development of forensic services over the next three to five years it should overcome any scarcity in placement opportunities. One respondent stated that and that the experience in secure environments should be optional.

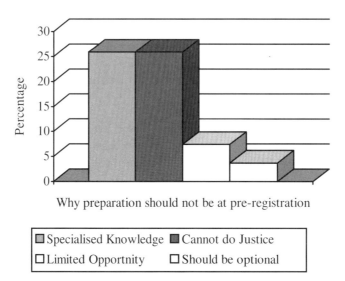

Why preparation should not be at pre-registration

- ▨ Specialised Knowledge ■ Cannot do Justice
- ☐ Limited Opportnity   ☐ Should be optional

Figure 13: Why preparation for working in a secure environment should not be at pre-registration

61 Education providers were asked what they felt the limitations were in offering preparation for students to work in secure environments. In all seven topic areas were identified by respondents (see figure 14) with three of these areas being identified by individual respondents.

62 The main area identified was in relation to time constraints which was mentioned by twelve respondents equalling 44 per cent. This again further supports the continuing theme from respondents of the pressures on the branch programmes of meeting a multiplicity of demands. The second area identified related to access to clinical placement where 11 respondents equalling 41 per cent mention this is a limitation. This somewhat contradicts responses to the earlier question on whether preparation should be at pre-registration when only one respondent cited this as an issue. However as previously mentioned problem of clinical placement should become less problematic with service developments in the coming few years.

63 Nine respondents cited inadequate teaching resources as a limitation (33 per cent) and this again confirms earlier responses in relation to numbers and recency of clinical experience of tutorial staff. As previously mentioned in relation to overcoming some

of these difficulties developments between service providers and education providers could resolve some of the inadequacy cited by respondents.

64   Three respondents (11 per cent) stated that students did not want placements in a secure environment and would support a view expressed in response to earlier questions of keeping this placement on an optional basis. A number of authors might suggest that as it is likely that all mental health services will increasingly have some patients presenting a multiplicity of problems including offending behaviours as well as more locally based secure environment and for education providers not to reflect this in a pre-registration curriculum would be unhelpful.

65   Single responses were received in relation to three topics. One referred to the role conflicts of working in secure environment particular in relation to security versus therapy and the lack of clarity about the goals of such services, particularly when some patients may not move on. Poor staff attitudes in secure environments were cited by one respondent and may reflect some local difficulties that they had experienced. One respondent referred to insufficient autonomy available for students in secure environment and may reflect the earlier comments in relation to higher staff numbers and richer skill mix and therefore more limited opportunity for students to take responsibility. This however would need to be counter balanced by the positive aspect of the availability of good supervision.

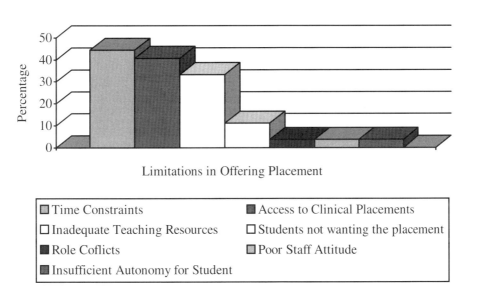

Figure 14: Limitations in offering preparation for students to work in secure environments

Main Themes and Concerns

66   Nursing in Secure Environments is a diverse concept, patients fit into all categories associated with branch programmes, i.e. Adult, Child, Mental Health and Learning Disabilities and are managed in a wide range of settings in the public and private sectors of health care and the Prison Service. There are many examples of good practice where attempts to enhance nursing provision and professional development are occurring, but from the work undertaken to date a number of recurring themes and concerns have emerged.

67   These themes and concerns are not only being voiced by practitioners and managers, but are also being raised by education providers. The methodologies that have been used, and the number of nurses contributing to the study validate the need for these issues to be addressed.

68   The main themes and concerns that are emerging from this work are as follows:

- time constraints and conflicting demands on pre-registration programmes both within the common foundation programme and the branch programmes

- availability and access to secure environments for placements

- lack of specific learning outcomes in relation to theory and practice for nursing in secure environments

- apparent lack of knowledge and understanding amongst education staff about services for patients in secure environments

- lack of research activity by educational establishments in relation to secure nursing care

- disparity of views as to whether this topic should be included in pre-registration or post registration nursing education programmes

- students emerge from nursing pre-registration programmes without the appropriate competencies to undertake the role of a registered practitioner

- service needs and cost constraints preclude effective preceptorship for newly qualified nurses

69   To address these issues and to provide guidance and support to nurses in secure environments a number of agencies and entities need to be involved. These include the National Boards for Nursing, Midwifery and Health Visiting, Education Commissioning Consortia, Educational Institutions, service providers within Health and the Prison Services both in the public and private sectors and staff side organisations.

References

Department of Health (1994) Report on working group on high security and related psychiatric provision (Chaired by Dr John Reed). London: Department of Health.

Department of Health (1998) Modernising Mental Health Services. London: Department of Health.

Department of Health and Social Security (1983) The Mental Health Act. London: DHSS.

Department of Health and Social Security (Northern Ireland) (1986) Mental Health (Northern Ireland) Act.

English National Board (1994) Creating Lifelong Learners- Partnership for Care. London: ENB.

Eraut M., Alderton, J., Boylan, A. and Wraight, A. (1995) An evaluation of the contribution of the biological and social sciences to pre-registration nursing and midwifery programmes. London: ENB.

May N, Veitch L McIntosh J, Alexander M (1997) Evaluation of Nurse and Midwife education in Scotland, 1992 programmes. Edinburgh: NBS.

McEvoy C (1995) The report of the summative evaluation of Project 2000 in Northern Ireland. Belfast: NBNI.

Mental Health Foundation (1998) Commissioning Services for Offenders with Mental Health Problems. London: Mental Health Foundation.

Polit D.F. and Hungler B.P. (1993) Essentials of Nursing Research: appraisal and utilisation. Philadelphia: J.B. Lippincot Company. pp 244-255.

Scottish Home and Health Department (1984) Mental Health (Scotland) Act.

Sainsbury Centre for Mental Health (1997) Pulling Together, the future roles and training of the mental health workforce. London: The Sainsbury Centre for Mental Health.

Les Storey and Colin Dale
Project Leaders
Nursing in Secure Environments Project

January 1999
paperedcomse

Bibliography

Anonymous (1993) Higher Education for Capability. *Capability News.*

Anonymous (1996) Mental Health Act is a bitter pill... arbitrary power of arrest. *Community Nurse.* 2, p8.

Anonymous (1998) Nurses left to sink or swim at Holloway. [Editorial comment]. *Mental Health Practice.*

Anonymous (1999) Nurses are at risk from inmates, say prison officers. *Nursing Times,* 95 edn, Vol. 22, p8.

Acheson, D. (1993) Comments on the Annual Report of the Director of Health Care. London: London School of Hygiene & Tropical Medicine.

Acheson, D. (1994) Commentary of the Health Advisory Committee on the Second Annual Report of the Director of Health Care Services for Prisoners. Department of Public Health and Policy.

Adebimpe, V.R. (1981) Overview: white norms and psychiatric diagnosis of black patients. *American Journal of Psychiatry*, 138, 279-285

Adler, N. (1997) Forensic Nursing. *Tar Heel Nurse.* 59, p35.

Adshead, G. (1994) Damage: Trauma and Violence in a Sample of Women Referred to a Forensic Service. *Behavioural Sciences and The Law.* 12, pp 235-249.

Adshead, G. (1997) "Written On The Body": Deliberate Self Harm And Violence. In: Welldon, E.V. and Van Velsen, C., (Eds.) *A Practical Guide To Forensic Psychotherapy*, Chap.14, pp 110-114. London: Jessica Kingsley Publications.

Agbolegbe, K. (1991) Psychiatric care for black patients. *Nursing Standard.* 5(45) pp37-39.

Aiyegbusi, A. (1997) Personality Disorder and Nursing at Ashworth Hospital [in The Written Submission to the Committee of Inquiry into the Personality Disorder Unit, Ashworth Hospital Authority].

Aiyegbusi, A. (1998) Clinical view. *Nursing Times.* p 94.

Alexander-Rodriguez, T. (1983) Prison health: a role for professional nursing. *Nursing Outlook.* 31(2) 115-118.

Allen, C. (1997) Asylum Seekers. *Nursing Times.* 93, pp 36-37.

Allen, D. (1991) Prison Nursing: Entering a very different world. *Nursing Standard.* 5(25) pp 22-23.

Allen, D. (1993) Prison Nursing: Doing time the hard way. *Nursing Standard.* 7(39) pp 20-22.

Alty, A. (1997) Nurses learning experience and expressed opinions regarding seclusion practice within one NHS trust. *Journal of Advanced Nursing.* 25.

American Nurses Association McHugh, J. and Leake, D., (Eds.) (1982) Standards of Psychiatric Nursing Practice. [Edited by McHugh, J. and Leake, D.] Washington: American Nurses Publishing.

American Nurses Association (1982) Standards of Psychiatric and Mental Health Practice. Kansas City, MO: American Nurses Publishing.

Australian Nursing Council Inc (1998) ANCI National Competency Standards for the Registered Nurse and the Enrolled Nurse. Australian Nursing Council Inc. Canberra

Asbury, J. (1995) Overview of Focus Group Research. *Qualitative Health Research*. 5 pp 414-420.

Ashworth Hospital Authority (1997) The Written Submission of Ashworth Hospital Authority by the Committee of Inquiry into the Personality Disorder Unit, Ashworth Hospital Authority.

Atkinson, J. (1991) Autonomy and Mental Health. In: Barker, P. and Baldwin, S., (Eds.) *Ethical Issues in Mental Health*. London: Churchill Livingstone.

Balajaran, R. (1991) Ethnic differences in mortality from ischaemic heart disease and cerebrovascular disease in England and Wales. *British Medical Journal*. pp 302, 560-564.

Barker, P. (1995) Psychiatry's human face. *Nursing Times*. 91, pp 58-59.

Barnard, K. (1980) Knowledge, Practice: Directions for the Future. *Nursing Research*. 29(4), pp 208-212.

Barnard, M. (1995) Stop this inhumane treatment of pregnant prisoners. [Letter] *Nursing Times*. (Dec. 6)

Barr, J. (1995) Pressure on nurses working in prison from non-qualified staff. [News] *Nursing Standard*. 9(45), p17.

Bartlett, A. (1993) What do we know about the English Special Hospitals? *International Journal of Law and Psychiatry*. 16.

Bavidge, M. (1989) *Mad or Bad?* Bristol: Bristol Classical Press.

Bazemore, G. and Liou, K.T. (1995) Lessons of Organisational Reform: a case study in policy change and staff impact in a secure detention facility. *Administration in Social Work*. 19(2), pp 25-45.

Bebbington, P.E., Feeney, S.T., Flannigan, C.B. and Glover, G.R. (1994) Inner London Collaborative Audit of Admissions in Two Health Districts: II. Ethnicity and the use of the Mental Health Act. *British Journal of Psychiatry*. 165(6), pp 743-749.

Beck, J.C. (1996) Forensic psychiatry in the USA and the. *Criminal Behaviour and Mental Health*. 6, pp 11-27.

Bellis, M.A., Weild, A.R., Beeching, N.J., Mutton, K.J. and Syed, Q. (1997) Prevalence of HIV and infecting drug use in men entering Liverpool prison. *British Medical Journal*. 315, pp 30-31.

Benner, P. (1984) *From Novice to Expert.* Menlo Park, California: Addison-Wesley.

Bernier, S.L. (1986) Corrections and mental health. *Journal of Psychosocial Nursing and Mental Health Services*. 24(6), pp 20-25.

Bhugra, D. (1997) Setting up psychiatric services: Cross-cultural issues in planning and delivery. *International Journal of Social Psychiatry*. 43, pp 16-28.

Bircumshaw, D. (1990) The utilisation of research findings in clinical nursing practice. *Journal of Advanced Nursing*. 15, pp 1272-1280.

Birmingham, L., Mason, D. and Grubin, D. (1996) Prevalence of mental disorder in remand prisoners: consecutive case study. *British Medical Journal*. 313, pp 1521-1524.

Black, J. and Laws, S. (1986) Living with sickle cell disease. London: Sickle Cell Society.

Blackburn, R. (1993) *The Psychology of Criminal Conduct.* Chichester: Wiley.

Blumstein, A. (1998) On the racial disproportionality of United States prisons. *Journal of Criminal Law and Criminology*. 73, pp 1259-1281.

Bondy, K.N., Jenkins, K., Seymour, L. and Lancaster, R. (1997) The development and testing of a competency-focused psychiatric nursing clinical evaluation instrument. *Archives of Psychiatric Nursing*. 11, pp 66-73.

Briant, S. and Freshwater, D. (1998) Exploring mutuality within the nurse-patient relationship. *British Journal of Nursing*. 7(4), pp 204-211.

Brimstead, A. Miller, A., and Robinson D (1998) Alternative therapy or good nursing care? Therapeutic touch with mentally disordered offenders. *Psychiatric Care*. 5(5) :pp 178-182

Browne, D. (1990) *Black people, mental health and the courts.* London: NACRO

Brooke, D., Taylor, C., Gunn, J. and Maden, A. (1996) Point prevalence of mental disorder in unconvicted male prisoners in England and Wales. *British Medical Journal*. 313, pp 1524-1527.

Brown, R.J. (1994) Forensic mental health. *Journal of Psychosocial Nursing and Mental Health Services*. 32, p10.

Browne, D.F. (1999) Developing Services for Mentally Disordered in Northern Ireland. Paper presented at the RCN 1st Annual Conference in Forensic Health Care Proceedings: 27 May 1999.

Bryman, A. and Cramer, D. (1997) *Quantitative Data Analysis with SPSS for Windows: A guide for social scientists.* London: Routledge.

Bullivant, M. (1996) A sense of justice... mentally disordered offenders, criminal justice system, liaison nursing. *Nursing Times.* 92, pp 44-45.

Bulmer C (1998) Clinical decisions:defining meaning through focus groups. *Nursing Standard.* 12(20), pp 34-36.

Bulmer, M.E. (1987) *Social Science and Social Policy.* London: Allen and Unwin.

Buncombe, A. (1998) McAliskey's mother to sue over detention. *The Independent.* Newspaper article: 11 Mar 1999.

Burrow, S. (1998) Therapy versus security: reconciling healing and damnation. In: Mason, T. and Mercer, D., (Eds.) *Critical perspectives in forensic care: inside out*, Chap.11, pp 171-187. London: McMillan Press Ltd.

Burrow, S. (1991) Mental Health: Special Hospitals - therapy versus custody. *Nursing Times.* 87 , pp 64-66.

Burrow, S. (1993) The role conflict of the forensic nurse... facilitating the health-management of the mentally abnormal offender. *Senior Nurse.* 13, pp 20-25.

Burrow, S. (1993) Inside the walls ... work of nursing staff in Special Hospitals and secure units. *Nursing Times.* 89, pp 38-40.

Burrow, S. (1993) The treatment and security needs of special-hospital patients: a nursing perspective. *Journal of Advanced Nursing.* 18, pp 1267-1278.

Burrow, S. (1994) Therapeutic security and the mentally-disordered offender. *British Journal of Nursing.* 3, pp 314-315.

Burrow, S. (1996) Special contribution... Special Hospitals, forensic nursing, high-security services. *Nursing Times.* 92, pp 54-56.

Burrows, R. (1995) Captive care: changes in prison nursing. *Nursing Standard.* 9, pp 29-31.

Butterworth, T. (1991) Generating Research in Mental Health Nursing. *International Journal of Nursing Studies.* 28(3), pp 237-246.

Butterworth, T. and Rushforth, D. (1995) Working in partnership with people who use services; reaffirming the foundations of practice for mental health nursing. *International Journal of Nursing Studies.* 32(4), pp 373-385.

Caddle, D.C.-D. (1997) Mothers in prison. *Home Office Research and Statistics Directorate.* No 38.

Calman, K.C. (1992) On the State of the Public Health 1991: The Annual Report of the Chief Medical Officer of the Department of Health for the year 1991. London: HMSO.

Calsin, J.B., Jr. (1992) Prison nursing: rising above fear to care. *Journal of Christ.Nursing.* 9(2), pp 22-26.

Campbell, L.S. (1994) Commentary on Violence. Edn. 4. p.14.

Carbonu, D.M. & Soares, J.M. (1997) Forensic nursing in Pakistan: Bridging the gap between victimised women and health care delivery systems. *Journal of Psychosocial Nursing and Mental Health Services* 35(6): pp 19-27

Carpenter, L. and Brockington, I.F. (1980) A Study of Mental Illness in Asians, West Indians and Africans living in Manchester. *British Journal of Psychiatry*, 137, pp 201-205

Carton, G. (1998) Nurse education: scribes and scriptures. In: MASON, T. and Mercer, D., (Eds.) *Critical perspectives in forensic care: inside out*, 1st edn. Chap.15, pp 244-255. London: McMillan Press Ltd.

Casedone, L.B. (1994) Go directly to jail... the Intervention Project for Nurses. *Nursingworld Journal*. 20(9), pp 1-24.

Castledine, G. (1998) Prison services are in urgent need of reform. *British Journal of Nursing*. p 616.

Catling P.C (1994) Mothers in prison. *Modern Midwife*. 4(6) pp 26-28.

Caton, C. (1981) The new chronic patient and the system of community care. *Hospital and Community Psychiatry*. 32 pp 475-478.

CCETSW (1995) Achieving Competence in Forensic Social Work. Pp 3-71. London: CCETSW.

Chaloner, C. (1998) Working in secure environments: ethical issues. *Mental Health Practice*. 2(2) pp 28-33.

Champion, V. and Leach, A. (1989) Variables related to Research Utilisation in Nursing: an empirical investigation. *Journal of Advanced Nursing*. 14 pp 705-710.

Chan, P. (1998) Paternalistic Interventions in Mental Health Care. *Nursing Times*. 94(36) pp 52-53.

Chanpakkee, J. and Whyte, L. (1996) Evaluating primary nursing in a secure environment. *Psychiatric Care*. 3 pp 188-193.

Cheater, F.M. and Closs, S.J. (1997) The effectiveness of methods of dissemination and implementation of clinical guidelines for nursing practice: a selective review. *Effectiveness in Nursing*. 1(1) pp 4-15.

Chen, E.Y.H., Harrison, G. and Standon, P. (1991) Management of the first episode of psychotic illness in Afro-Caribbean patients. British Journal of Psychiatry, 158 pp 517-522

Chiswick, D. (1993) Forensic Psychiatry. In: Kendall, R.E. and Zealley, A.K., (Eds.) *Companion to Psychiatric Studies*. Edinburgh: Churchill Livingstone.

Chiswick, D. and Dooley E (1995) Psychiatry in Prisons. In Chiswick D, Cope E (eds) Practical Forensic Psychiatry. London: Gaskell, pp 243-271

Clark, J. (1993) The Future of Nurse Education. Report of the RCN Consensus Conference. Sept 1993. London: RCN.

Clarke, A. and Jack, B. (1998) The benefits of using qualitative research. *Nurse*.

Clarke, L. (1995) Psychiatric nursing and electroconvulsive therapy. *Nursing International Journal for Health Care Professionals*. 2, pp 321-331.

Clarke, L. (1996) Participant Observation in a Secure Unit: care, conflict and control. *Nursing Times research*. 1(6) pp 431-441.

Clarke, L. (1997) Flowers in their mouths. *Changes*. p117.

Clinical Resource and Audit Group (1993) Clinical Guidelines: A Report by a Working Group Set Up by the Clinical Resource and Audit Group. Edinburgh: Scottish Office.

Coffey, M. (1997) Mental Health Nursing. Supervised discharge: concerns about the new powers for nurses. *British Journal of Nursing*. 6, pp 215-218.

Cohen, A. and Eastman, N. (1997) Needs Assessment for Mentally Disordered Offenders and Others Requiring Similar Services. *British Journal of Psychiatry*. p 171.

Cohen, A. and Eastman, N. (1997) Minimum Secure Services in South West Thames: a description of operational policies and patient characteristics. *Journal of Forensic Psychiatry*. p100.

Coles, J. (1998) Is justice really served by tearing this baby from her mother's arms? *The Express*. Newspaper article: 12 Nov 1998.

Coll, C.G., Miller, J.B., Fields, J.P. and Mathews, B. (1997) The Experiences of Women in Prison: Implications for services and prevention. *Women and Therapy*. 20, pp 11-28.

Collins, M. and Robinson, D. (1997) Studying Patient Choice and Privacy in a Forensic Setting. *Psychiatric Care*. 4, (1) pp 12-15.

Collins, M. and Robinson, D. (1997) Measuring aggression in forensic psychiatric care. *Psychiatric Care*. 4,(2) pp 67 70

Conroy, M. (1996) The Future Health Care Workforce. Manchester University: HSMU.

Consedine, M. (1998) Paper presented at the First New Zealand Child and Youth Mental Health Conference: "Today's Tomorrow - The Mental Health of our Tamariki and Rangatahi". Christchurch: ANZCMHN.

[Available http://homepages.ihug.co.nz/-chattan/clinsup1.htm].

Coombes, R. (1996) From Carers to Custodians. *Nursing Times*. p19.

Cope R (1989) The compulsory detention of Afro-Caribbeans under the Mental Health Act New Community, 13(3), pp 343-356.

Coram, J.W. (1993) Forensic Nurse Specialists; working with Perpetrators and hostage negotiation teams. *Journal of Psychosocial nursing* 31(11) pp 26-30

Cornah, D., Stein, K. and Stevens, A. (1997) The Therapeutic Community Method of Treatment for Borderline Personality Disorder.

Covington, S. (1998) Women in prison: Approaches in the treatment of our most invisible population. *Women and Therapy.* 21, pp 141-155.

Crabbe, G. (1988) Care or Control? *Nursing Times.* 84(28), p19.

Crane, J. (1985) Using Research in Practice, Research Utilisation: Theoretical Perspectives. *Western Journal of Nursing Research.* 7(2), pp 261-268.

Crichton, J. (1997) Response of nursing staff to psychiatric patient misdemeanour. *Journal of Forensic Psychiatry.* p61.

Crimlisk, H. and Phelan, M. (1995) "Reform of the Mental Health Act 1983: An effective tribunal system?" [Comment]. *British Journal of Psychiatry.* 167(1), pp 116-117.

Crowley, J.J. and Simmons, S. (1992) Mental health, race and ethnicity: a retrospective study of the care of ethnic minorities and whites in a psychiatric unit. *Journal of Advanced Nursing.* 17(9), pp 1078-1087.

Cruickshank, J.K., Beevers, D.G., Osbourne, V.L., Haynes, R.A., Corlett, J.C.R. and Selby, S. (1980) Heart attack, stroke, diabetes and hypertension in West Indians, Asians, and whites in Birmingham, England. *British Medical Journal.* 281, p1108.

Curran, C., Grimshaw, C., Zigmond, A. and Milligan, A. (1997) Mental Health Act. A brief guide to the 1983 Act. Part III. *Psychiatric Care.* 4, pp 39-42.

Cutcliffe, J.R. (1998) What direction for mental health research? *British Journal of Nursing.* 7 (10), p 570.

Dale, C., Rae, M. and Tarbuck, P. (1995) Changing the culture in a Special Hospital. *Nursing Times.* 91(30), pp 33-35.

Dale, C., Wallis, E. and Taylor, J. (1999) Professional, contractual and volunteer relationships. In: Taylor, P. and Swan, T., (Eds.) *Couples in care and custody,* Chap.13, pp 159-187. Oxford: Butterworth Heinemann.

Dale, C. (1990) Introduction to Quality Assurance. *Nursing Times.* 4(21).

Davis, B.D. (1981) Trends in psychiatric nursing research. *Nursing Times.* 77(26).

Davis, B.D. (1986) A review of recent research in psychiatric nursing. *British Journal of Nursing.* 4(21).

Davis, B.D. (1990) Research and psychiatric nursing. *British Journal of Nursing.* 4(21).

Day, C. (1983) The Challenge: Health Care vs. Security. *The Canadian Nurse.* 79(7), pp 34-36.

Dean, G. Walsh, D and Downing H. (1981) First admissions of Native Born and Immigrants to Psychiatric Hospitals in South-East England, 1970. British Journal of Psychiatry, 139, pp 506-512.

Department of Health (1974)   Revised report of the working party on security in NHS psychiatric hospitals (The Glancy Report). London: HMSO.

Department of Health and Social Security (1983) The Mental Health Act. London: DHSS.

Department of Health and Social Security (Northern Ireland) (1986) Mental Health (North Ireland) Act. DHSS (Northern Ireland).

Department of Health (1992) Report of the committee of inquiry into complaints about Ashworth Hospital. (The Blom-Cooper Report). London: HMSO

Department of Health (1992) Review of health and social services for mentally disordered offenders and others requiring similar services. Services for people from black and ethnic minority groups. Issues of race and culture. Home Office.

Department of Health (1992) Executive Letter. EL(92)24. Leeds: NHS Executive.

Department of Health (1994)   Report of working group on high security and related psychiatric provision. (Chaired by Dr John Reed). London: Department of Health.

Department of Health (1994) Working in Partnership: Review of the Mental Health Nursing Review Team. London: HMSO.

Department of Health (1994) *Black mental health- a dialogue for change.* NHS Mental Health Task Force. London: Department of Health

Department of Health (1995) *Black mental health- a dialogue for change.*   Wetherby Department of Health

Department of Health (1995) Methods to Promote The Implementation of Research Findings in The NHS: Priorities for Evaluation. London: HMSO.

Department of Health National Health Management Executive, (Ed.) (1996)   Promoting clinical effectiveness: a framework for action in and through the NHS.   Leeds: Department of Health.

Department of Health (1998)   Modernising Mental Health Services: Safe, Sound and Supportive. London: HMSO.

Department of Health (1999) Review of prescribing, supply & administration of medicines. Final Report. London: Department of Health.

Department of Health (1999) Safer Services: National Confidential Inquiry into Suicide and Homicide by People with Mental Illness. London: Department of Health

Department of Health and Social Security (1972)   Report of the Committee on Mentally Abnormal Offenders (The Butler Report). CMND6244. London: DHSS.

Department of Social Services (1998) Modernising Social Services. London: The Stationery Office.

Devlin, A. (1998) *Invisible women.   What's wrong with women's prisons?*   1st edn. Waterside Press.

Dhondea, R. (1995) An ethnographic study of nurses in a forensic psychiatric setting: education and training implications. *Australian New Zealand Journal of Mental Health Nursing.* 4, pp 77-82.

Dilorio, C.et al. (1994) Focus groups: an interview message for nursing research. *Journal of neuroscience nursing.* 26(3), pp 175-180.

Dimond, B. (1999) Pregnant women in prison and the law on human rights. *British Journal of Midwifery.* 7(5), pp 297-299.

Doku, J. (1998) Approaches to cultural awareness. *Nursing Times.*

Dolan, B. and Coid, J. (1993) *Psychopathic and Antisocial Disorders: Treatment and Research issues.* London: Gaskell.

Dolan, B. and Bland, J. (1996) Who are the women in special hospitals? In: Hemingway, C., (Ed.) *Special Women?: The experience of women in the Special Hospital system..* Aldershot: Avebury.

Dolan, J. (1998) Self-harm in the Prison Environment. *Prison Service Journal.* 118, pp 11-13.

Donaldson, L.J. and Taylor, J.B. (1983) Patterns of Asians and non-Asians morbidity in hospitals. *British Medical Journal.* 286, pp 949-951.

Donnelly, M (1983) Managing the mind: A study of medical psychology in early nineteenth century Britain. London: Tavistock

Drake, R.E., Osher, F.C. and Wallach, M.A. (1989) Alcohol use and abuse in schizophrenia: a prospective community study. *Journal of Nervous and Mental Disease.* 177, pp 408-414.

Drake, R.E., Rosenberg, S.D. and Mueser, K.T. (1996) Assessing substance use disorder in persons with severe mental illness. In: Drake, R.E. and Mueser, K.T., (Eds.) *Dual diagnosis of major mental illness and substance abuse,* pp 3-17. San Francisco: Jossey-Bass.

Drake, V.K. (1998) Process, perils, and pitfalls of research in prison. *Issues in Mental Health Nursing.* 19, pp 41-52.

Droes, N. (1994) Correctional Nursing Practice. *Journal of Community Health.* 11(4), pp 201-210.

Droes, N.S. (1931) An exploration of the nature and problems of nursing practice in correctional settings. p.317 University of California, San Francisco: DNS.

Droes, N.S. (1994) Correctional nursing practice. *Journal of Community Health Nursing.* 11(4), pp 201-210.

Duff, A. (1996) Case study of a female client on a regional secure unit. *Journal of Advanced Nursing.* 23(4), pp 771-775.

Duff, L.A., Kitson, A.L., Seers, K. and Humphris, D. (1996) Clinical Guidelines: an introduction to their development and implementation. *Journal of Advanced Nursing.* 23, pp 887-895.

Duffy, D., Clifton, M. and Dale, C. (1997) Mental health inquiry reports: the lessons for nursing. *Mental Health Practice.* p16.

Dulfer, S. (1992) No Holds Barred. *Nursing.* 5(4), pp 20-22.

Dunn, W. (1983) Measuring knowledge use. *Knowledge, Creation, Diffusion & Utilisation.* 1(1), pp 477-498.

Edwards, S. (1992) Perspectives on race and gender. In Stockdale, E. Casale, S.(eds) Criminal Justice Under Stress, pp 246-264. London: Blackstone Press.

Elliott, R.L. (1997) Evaluating the quality of correctional mental health services: An approach to surveying a correctional mental health system. *Behavioural Sciences and the Law.* 15 pp 427-438.

English National Board (1994) Creating Lifelong Learners - Partnership for Care. London: ENB.

Epstein, R. and Simon.R. (1990) The Exploitation Index: an early viewing indicator of boundary violations in psychotherapy. pp 450-465.

Eraut, M. and Cole, G. (1993) Assessing competence in the professions. Report no. 14. Sheffield: Department of Employment.

Eraut, M., Alderton, J., Boylan, A. and Wraight, A. (1995) An evaluation of the contribution of the biological and social sciences to pre-registration nursing and midwifery programmes. London: ENB.

Evans, A. and McGilvray, L. (1996) RN's trial a forensic nursing service. *Australian Journal of Advanced Nursing.* 14, pp 11-15.

Evan, A and Wells, D (1999) An exploration of the role of the Australian Forensic Nurse. Royal College of Nursing, Australia.

Evans, K. and Sullivan, J.M. (1990) *Dual diagnosis: Counselling the mentally ill substance abuser.* New York: Guilford.

Fallon, P., Bluglass, R., Edwards, B. and Daniels, G. (1999) Report of the Committee of Inquiry into the Personality Disorder Unit, Ashworth Special Hospital. Volume II. Expert Evidence on Personality Disorder. 'The Fallon Report'. London: The Stationery Office.

Farrington, A. (1993) Transcultural psychiatry, ethnic minorities and marginalization. *British Journal of Nursing.* 2(16), pp 805-809.

Faulk M (1994) Psychopathic disorder and forensic psychiatry. In: Anonymous *Basic Forensic Psychiatry*, 2nd edn. Chap.10, pp 193-212. Blackwell Science Ltd.

Faulk M (1994) Ethics and forensic psychiatry. In: Anonymous *Basic Forensic Psychiatry*, 2nd edn. Chap.16, pp 315-331. Blackwell Science Ltd.

Faulk M (1994) Management of patients within secure psychiatric institutions. In: Anonymous *Basic Forensic Psychiatry*, 2nd edn. Chap.17, pp 332-351. Blackwell Science Ltd.

Feeg, V.D. (1998) Solving health problems with treatment, not jail. *Pediatric Nursing*. 18(1), p 8.

Feehan, C.J. (1994) Audit of the use of the Mental Health Act in a psychogeriatric hospital. *International Journal of Geriatric Psychiatry*. 9(7), pp 563-565.

Fergusson, S., McComish, A. and Paterson, B. (1997) Clinical outcome measures: psychopathy - a developmental framework. *Psychiatric Care*. 4, pp 71-74.

Fernando, S., Ndegwa, D. and Wilson, M. (1998) *Forensic Psychiatry, Race and Culture.* London: Routledge.

Ferns, P. and Madden, M. (1998) Training to promote race equality. In: Fernando, S., (Ed.) *Mental health in a multi ethnic society.*

Firth-Cozens, J. (1997) Healthy promotion: changing behaviour towards evidence based health care. *Quality in Health Care*. 6, pp 205-211.

Fish, D. and Purr, B. (1991) An evaluation of practice based learning. In: English National Board, (Ed.) *Continuing Professional Education in Nursing, Midwifery and Health Visiting. Project Paper 4.* London: English National Board (ENB).

Fisher, A. (1995) The ethical problems encountered in psychiatric nursing practice with dangerous mentally ill persons. *Scholarly Inquiry for Nursing Practice*. 9, pp 193-208.

Fitzpatrick, J.M., While, A.E. and Roberts, J.D. (1996) Operationalisation of an observation instrument to explore nurse performance. *International Journal of Nursing Studies*. 33, pp 349-360.

Flemming, K. (1998) Asking answerable questions. *Evidence Based Nursing*. Apr 98. (2).

Ford, J. and Rigby, P. (1996) Focus on mental health nursing. Aftercare under supervision: implications for CMHN's. *British Journal of Nursing*. 5, pp 1312-1316.

Ford, K. (1997) Primary health care workers; training needs in mental health. *British Journal of Nursing*.

Francis, E. (1996) Community care, danger and Black People. *OPENMIND*, 80, pp 4-5

Freemantle, N., Grillo, R., Grimshaw, J. and Oxman, A. (1995) Implementing findings of medical research: The Cochrane Collaboration on Effective Professional Practice. *Quality in Health Care*. 4, pp 45-47.

Fulop, N.J. (1995) Supervised discharge: lessons from the US experience. *Mental Health Nursing*. 15, pp 16-20.

Funk, S., Champayne, M. and Wiese, R. (1991) Barriers to Using Research Findings in Practice: The Clinician's Perspective. *Applied Nursing Research.* 4, pp 90-95.

Gadd, D., McFadden, K. and Colgan, L. (1995) *Research Based Care Planning: A case study of research use by mental health nurses.* Manchester: Cartmel NDU.

Gallop, R. (1997) Abuse of power in the nurse client relationship: definition, research and organisational response. Paper presented at UKCC Conference. Summer 1997.

Geddes, N., Mark, B.A. and Salyer, J. (1997) Outcomes Research: clues to quality and organisational effectiveness. *Nursing Clinics of North America.* Sept 97. 32(3), pp 589-601.

Gelder, M.G. (1998) A Core Curriculum in Psychiatry for Medical Students. *Current Opinion in Psychiatry.* 11(5), pp 491-502.

George, S. (1998) More than a pound of flesh: a patient's perspective. In: Mason, T. and Mercer, D., (Eds.) *Critical perspectives in forensic care: inside out,* Chap.7, pp 102-107. London: McMillan Press.

Gillon, R. (1985) *Philosophical Medical Ethics.* Chichester: Wiley.

Gillon, R. (1996) Thinking about a medical school core curriculum for medical ethics and law. *Journal of Medical Ethics.* 22, pp 323-324.

Gilmore, A. (1998) Impact Evaluation of Professional Standards. [Unpublished document].

Gilmore, C., Wood, G.C. and Rigby, J.C. (1994) Elderly patients and the Mental Health Act 1983. *International Journal of Geriatric Psychiatry.* 9(10), pp 809-818.

Gournay, K. (1995) Mental health nurses working purposefully with people with serious and enduring mental illness - an international perspective. *International Journal of Nursing Studies.* 32(4), pp 341-352.

Gray, R., Smedley, N. and Thomas, B. (1997) The use of Section 136: A review of research 1972-96. *Psychiatric Care.* 4, pp 62-66.

Gray, R. and Thomas, B. (1998) Violent behaviour and locked wards: a review of effects on patients. *Journal of Interpersonal Violence.* P 411.

Greenbaum, T.L. (1998) *The Handbook for Focus Group Research.* 2nd edn. London: Sage.

Grimshaw, J. and Russell, I. (1993) Effect of clinical guidelines on medical practice: a systematic review of rigorous evaluations. *The Lancet.* 342, pp 1317-1322.

Grimshaw, J. and Russell, I. (1993) Achieving health gain through clinical guidelines. 1: Developing scientifically valid guidelines. *Quality in Health Care.* 2, pp 245-248.

Grimshaw, J. and Russell, I. (1994) Achieving health gain through clinical guidelines. 11: Ensuring guidelines change medical practice. *Quality in Health Care.* 3, pp 45-52.

Grimshaw, J., Freemantle, N., Wallace, S., Russell, I., Hurwitz, B., Watt, I., Long, A. and Sheldon, T. (1995) Developing and implementing clinical practice guidelines. *Quality in Health Care.* 4 , pp 45-52.

Grol, R. (1992) Implementing guidelines in general practice care. *Quality in Health Care.* 1, pp 184-191.

Grubin, D. (1993) Services for mentally disordered offenders. *Criminal Behaviour and Mental Health.* 3, pp 3-6.

Gulland, A. (1997) A special legacy of neglect. [Editorial comment]. *Nursing Times.* 93, pp 16-17.

Gulland, A. (1998) It's purely professional. *Nursing Times.* 94, pp 12-13.

Gulland, A. (1998) Mental health crisis in the capital. *Nursing Times.* 94, p 19.

Gulotta, K. (1987) Factors Affecting Nursing Practice in a Correctional Health Care Setting. *Journal of Prison and Jail Health.* 6(1), pp 3-22.

Gunn, J., Maden, A. and Swinton, J. (1991) Treatment needs of prisoners with psychiatric disorders. *British Medical Journal.* 303, pp 338-341.

Gunn, J. (1999) Written submission to Report of the Committee of Inquiry into the Personality Disorder Unit, Ashworth Special Hospital. Volume II: Expert Evidence on Personality Disorder. Department of Health. London: The Stationery Office.

Gutheil, T.G. and Gabbard, G.O. (1993) The concept of boundaries in clinical practice: theoretical and risk management dimensions. *American Journal of Psychiatry.* 150, pp 180-196.

Habermas, J. (1991) The theory of communicative action, reason and the rationalisation of society (Volume 1). Translated [from the German] Thomas McCarthy. *Clinical Effectiveness in Nursing.* 2, pp 86-93.

Haigh, R. and Clarke, L. (1995) Commentary: "An examination of therapeutic principles and practice in two forensic units". *Journal of Psychiatric and Mental Health Nursing.* 2, pp 187-189.

Haines, G. (1997) Mental Health Education: Where to now? *Nursing Times.* 93, pp 61-63.

Henderson, S. and Robinson, D. (1997) Developing a behavioural status index to assess patient dangerousness. Mental Health Care. 1(4) : pp 130-132

Hall, R.C., Beresford, T.P., Gardner, E.R. and Popkin, M.K. (1982) The medical care of psychiatric patients. *Hospital and Community Psychiatry.* 31, pp 463-472.

Hamill, C. and McAleer, J. (1996) Analysing qualitative data using a software package. *Nursing Researcher.*

Harrison, A. (1997) Consent and common law. *Nursing Times.* 93, pp 52-54.

Harrison, G., Ineichen, B. and Morgan, H.G. (1984) Psychiatric Hospital Admissions in Bristol. (1) Geographic and Ethnic factors. (2) Social and Clinical factors of compulsory admissions. *British Journal of Psychiatry*, 145, pp 60-0-611

Heinze, M.C. (1997) Borderline personality disorder and forensic mental health. *Journal of the California Alliance for the Mentally Ill*. 8, pp 22-24.

Hemingway, C. (1996) *Special Women? The experience of women in the Special Hospital system*. Aldershot: Avebury.

Herman, J.L. (1992) *Trauma And Recovery: From Domestic Violence To Political Terror*. London: Basic Books.

Higgins, J. (1996) Future of the Special Hospitals. *Criminal Behaviour and Mental Health*. (Suppl), pp 65-72.

Hill, J.B. (1993) County jail health care services: summary of findings. *Florida Nurse*. 41(10),pp 8-9.

Hinton, P.R. (1995) *Statistics explained: a guide for social science students*. London: Routledge.

HM Chief Inspector of Prisons for England and Wales (1996) HM Prison Manchester. Jan. London: Home Office.

HM Chief Inceptor of Prisons for England and Wales (1997) HM Prison Dartmoor. 3-7 Nov. London: Home Office.

HM Chief Inspector of Prisons for England and Wales (1997) HM Prison Lewes (Part B). 7-12 Sept. London: Home Office.

HM Chief Inspector of Prisons for England and Wales (1997) HM Prison Holloway. 8-12 Dec. London: Home Office.

HM Chief Inspector of Prisons for England and Wales (1997) HM Prison Wakefield. 10-18 Nov. London: Home Office.

HM Chief Inspector of Prisons for England and Wales (1997) Tinsley House Immigration Detention Centre Gatwick Airport (Part A - Executive Summary). 4-7 Aug. London: Home Office.

HM Chief Inspector of Prisons for England and Wales (1997) Tinsley House Immigration Detention Centre Gatwick Airport (Part B - Main Report). 4-7 Aug. London: Home Office.

HM Chief Inspector of Prisons for England and Wales (1998) HM Prison Everthorpe. 18-22 May. London: Home Office.

HM Chief Inspector of Prisons for England and Wales (1998) HM Prison Birmingham. 7-9 Sept. London: Home Office.

HM Chief Inspector of Prisons for England and Wales (1998) Campsfield House Detention Centre. 13-15 Oct. London: Home Office.

HM Chief Inspector of Prisons for England and Wales (1998) HM Prison Winchester. 9-13 Feb. London: Home Office.

HM Chief Inspector of Prisons for England and Wales (1998) HM Prison The Wolds. 2-6 Nov. London: Home Office.

HM Chief Inspector of Prisons for England and Wales (1998) HM Prison and Young Offender Institution Hindley. 14-15 Dec. London: Home Office.

HM Chief Inspector of Prisons for England and Wales (1998) HM Holding Centre Haslar. 15-19 Jun. London: Home Office.

HM Chief Inspector of Prisons for England and Wales (1998) HM Prison Woodhill. 14-16 Jul. London: Home Office.

HM Chief Inspector of Prisons for England and Wales (1998) HM Prison Chelmsford. 20-22 Oct. London: Home Office.

HM Chief Inspector of Prisons for England and Wales (1998) HM Prison Stafford. 12-14 May. London: Home Office.

HM Chief Inspector of Prisons for England and Wales (1998) HM Prison and Young Offender Institution Askham Grange. 12-16 Oct. London: Home Office.

HM Chief Inspector of Prisons for England and Wales (1998) HM Prison Nottingham. 29 Jun-3 Jul. London: Home Office.

HM Chief Inspector of Prisons for England and Wales (1998) HM Prison and Young Offender Institution Doncaster. 3-5 Nov. London: Home Office.

HM Chief Inspector of Prisons for England and Wales (1998) HM Prison Highpoint. 29 Jun-1 Jul. London: Home Office.

HM Chief Inspector of Prisons for England and Wales (1998) HM Prison North Sea Camp. 27-29 Jul. London: Home Office.

HM Chief Inspector of Prisons for England and Wales (1998) HM Prison Bedford. 27 Apr-1 May. London: Home Office.

HM Chief Inspector of Prisons for England and Wales (1998) HM Prison The Maze. 23 Mar-3 Apr. London: Home Office.

HM Chief Inspector of Prisons for England and Wales (1998) HM Prison Lewes (Part A - Executive Summary). 7-12 Sept. London: Home Office.

HM Chief Inspector of Prisons for England and Wales (1998) HM Prison Lewes (Part B - Main Report). 7-12 Sept. London: Home Office.

HM Chief Inspector of Prisons for England and Wales (1998) HM Young Offender Institution and Remand Centre Feltham. 30 Nov-4 Dec.

HM Chief Inspector of Prisons for England and Wales (1998) HM Prison Leicester. 5-9 Oct. London: Home Office.

HM Chief Inspector of Prisons for England and Wales (1998) HM Prison Kirkham. 13-18 Sept. London: Home Office.

HM Chief Inspector of Prisons for England and Wales (1998) HM Young Offender Institution Aylesbury. 8-12 Jun. London: Home Office.

HM Chief Inspector of Prisons for England and Wales (1998) HM Prison Belmarsh. 11-20 May. London: Home Office.

HM Chief Inspector of Prisons for England and Wales (1998) HM Prison Sudbury. 13-17 Jul. London: Home Office.

HM Chief Inspector of Prisons for England and Wales (1998) HM Prison Blakenhurst. 5-7 Oct. London: Home Office.

HM Chief Inspector of Prisons for England and Wales (1998) HM Prison Albany. 30 Sept-1 Oct. London: Home Office.

HM Chief Inspector of Prisons for England and Wales (1998) HM Prison Long Lartin. 20-28 Apr. London: Home Office.

HM Chief Inspector of Prisons for England and Wales (1998) HM Prison Gloucester. 30 Mar-1 Apr. London: Home Office.

HM Chief Inspector of Prisons for England and Wales (1998) HM Prison Frankland. 5-13 Jan. London: Home Office.

HM Chief Inspector of Prisons for England and Wales (1998) HM Prison Norwich. 27-30 Jul. London: Home Office.

HM Chief Inspector of Prisons for England and Wales (1998) HM Prison Wellingborough. 2-6 Mar. London: Home Office.

HM Chief Inspector of Prisons for England and Wales (1998) HM Prison The Mount. 16-20 Mar. London: Home Office.

HM Chief Inspector of Prisons for England and Wales (1999) HM Prison Lincoln. 11-15 Jan. London: Home Office.

HM Chief Inspector of Prisons for England and Wales (1999) HM Prison Blakenhurst. 5-7 Oct. London: Home Office.

HM Chief Inspector of Prisons for England and Wales (1996) HM Prison Chelmsford (Part B). 30 Sept-4 Oct. London: Home Office.

HM Chief Inspector of Prisons for England and Wales (1996) HM Prison/Young Offenders Institution Drake Hall (Part B). 2-6 Dec. London: Home Office.

HM Chief Inspector of Prisons for England and Wales (1996) HM Young Offenders Institution and Remand Centre Feltham (Part B). 28 Oct-5 Nov. London: Home Office.

HM Chief Inspector of Prisons for England and Wales (1996) HM Prison Gloucester. 15-19 Jul. London: Home Office.

HM Chief Inspector of Prisons for England and Wales (1996) HM Prison Lancaster. London: Home Office.

HM Chief Inspector of Prisons for England and Wales (1996) HM Prison Styal. 3-8 Nov. London: Home Office.

HM Chief Inspector of Prisons for England and Wales (1996) HM Prison The Verne. London: Home Office.

HM Chief Inspector of Prisons for England and Wales (1996) HM Prison Holloway. Unannounced inspection. London: Home Office.

HM Chief Inspector of Prisons for England and Wales (1997) Women in Prison: A thematic review. London: Home Office.

HM Chief Inspector of Prisons for England and Wales (1997) Young Prisoners: A thematic review. London: Home Office.

HM Chief Inspector of Prisons for England and Wales (1997) HM Prison Aldington (Part B). 14-18 Apr. London: Home Office.

HM Chief Inspector of Prisons for England and Wales (1997) HM Prison Buckley Hall (Part B). 10-14 Feb. London: Home Office.

HM Chief Inspector of Prisons for England and Wales (1997) HM Prison Canterbury (Part B). 29 Sept-3 Oct. London: Home Office.

HM Chief Inspector of Prison for England and Wales (1997) HM Prison Cookham Wood. 27-31 Oct. London: Home Office.

HM Chief Inspector of Prisons for England and Wales (1997) HM Prison Erlestoke. 6-11 Jul. London: Home Office.

HM Chief Inspector of Prisons for England and Wales (1997) HM Prison Full Sutton. 6-16 Jan. London: Home Office.

HM Chief Inspector of Prisons for England and Wales (1997) HM YOI Glen Parva. Unannounced inspection: 1-5 Dec. London: Home Office.

HM Chief Inspector of Prisons for England and Wales (1997) HM Prisons Grendon and Springhill (Part B). 1-12 Sept. London: Home Office.

HM Chief Inspector of Prison for England and Wales (1997) HM Prison Holloway. Unannounced inspection: 8-12 Dec. London: Home Office.

HM Chief Inspector of Prisons for England and Wales (1997) HM Prison North Sea Camp. London: Home Office.

HM Chief Inspector of Prisons for England and Wales (1997) HM Prison Swaleside (Part B). 3-7 Feb. London: Home Office.

HM Chief Inspector of Prisons for England and Wales (1997) HM Prison Wealstun (Part B). 14-18 Jul. London: Home Office.

HM Chief Inspector of Prison for England and Wales (1998) HM Prison Featherstone. 26-30 Jan. London: Home Office.

HM Chief Inspector of Prisons for England and Wales (1998) HM Prison The Mount. 16-20 Mar. London: Home Office.

HM Chief Inspector of Prisons for England and Wales (1998) HM Prison Wellingborough. 2-6 Mar. London: Home Office.

HM Chief Inspector of Prisons for England and Wales (1998) HM Prison Winchester. 9-13 Feb. London: Home Office.

HM Inspectorate of Prisons for England & Wales (1996) Patient or prisoner? A new strategy for health care in prisons. London: Home Office.

HM Inspectorate of Prisons for England & Wales (1998) Annual Report of HM Chief Inspector of Prisons for England & Wales 1997-1998. London: The Stationery Office Limited.

HM Inspectorate of Prisons for England and Wales (1998) HM Prison The Verne. 21-22 Apr. London: Home Office.

HM Inspectorate of Prisons for England and Wales (1998) HM Prison Elmley. 17-19 Nov. London: Home Office.

HM Inspectorate of Prisons & Probation (1999) Lifers. London: Home Office.

HM Inspectorate of Prisons for Scotland (1996) HM Prison Castle Huntly. Edinburgh : Scottish Office

HM Inspectorate of Prisons for Scotland (1996) HM Prison Cornton Vale. Edinburgh : Scottish Office

HM Inspectorate of Prisons for Scotland (1996) HM Prison Edinburgh. Edinburgh : Scottish Office

HM Inspectorate of Prisons for Scotland (1996) HM Prison Glenochil. Edinburgh : Scottish Office

HM Inspectorate of Prisons for Scotland (1997) HM Prison Aberdeen. Edinburgh : Scottish Office

HM Inspectorate of Prisons for Scotland (1997) HM Prison Barlinnie. Edinburgh : Scottish Office

HM Inspectorate of Prisons for Scotland (1997) HM Prison Longriggend. Edinburgh : Scottish Office

HM Inspectorate of Prisons for Scotland (1997) HM Prison Penninghame. Edinburgh : Scottish Office

HM Inspectorate of Prisons for Scotland (1997) HM Prison Perth. Edinburgh : Scottish Office

HM Inspectorate of Prisons for Scotland (1998) HM Prison Low Moss. Edinburgh : Scottish Office

HM Inspectorate of Prisons for Scotland (1998) HM National Induction Centre. Edinburgh : Scottish Office

HM Inspectorate of Prisons for Scotland (1998) HM Prison Noranside. Edinburgh : Scottish Office

HM Inspectorate of Prisons for Scotland (1998) HM Young Offenders Institution Polmont. Edinburgh : Scottish Office

HM Inspectorate of Prisons for Scotland (1998) HM Prison Shotts. Edinburgh : Scottish Office

HM Inspectorate of Prisons for Scotland (1999) HM Prison Inverness. Edinburgh : Scottish Office

HM Prison Service (1998) Annual Report of the Director of Health Care. London: The Stationery Office.

HM Prison Service and NHS Executive (1999) The Future Organisation of Prison Health Care. Report of the Joint Prison Service and National Health Service Executive Working Group. London: Department of Health.

Hogston, R. (1993) From competent novice to competent expert: a discussion of competence in the light of post registration and practice project (PREPP). *Nurse Education Today*. 13(3), pp 341-344.

Holleran, C. (1983) Ethics in prison health care. *International Nursing Review*. 30(5), pp 138-140.

Holmberg, S. (1988) Physical health problems of the psychiatric client. *Journal of Psychosocial Nursing and Mental Health Services*. 26(5), pp 35-39.

Holmes, C.A. (1991) Psychopathic Disorder: a category mistake? *Journal of Medical Ethics* 17: 77-85

Holmes, C.A. (1997) On 'not caring' in forensic settings. Paper presented at Mental Health and the Millenium- Difficult decisions in Dangerous Worlds: 6th Congress on Mental Health Nursing. London, October 8-10

Home Office (1964) Prison Rules Act. London: HMSO.

Home Office (1991) Standing Order 13: Health Care. London: HMSO.

Home Office (1993) Prison Service Annual Report & Accounts. April 1992-March 1993. London: HMSO.

Horsley, J., Crane, J., Crabtree, M.K. and Wood, D.J. (1983) *Using Research to Improve Practice: A Guide.* New York: Grune & Stratton.

House of Commons (1985) Third Report from the Social Services Committee Session 1985-86 on Prison Medical Services. London: HMSO.

Huckle, P.L. (1997) The use of patient satisfaction surveys in forensic psychiatric settings. *Psychiatric Care.* 4, pp 230-233.

Hunt, J. (1981) Indicators for nursing practice: the use of research findings. *Journal of Advanced Nursing.* 6, pp 189-194.

Hunt, M. (1987) The Process of Translating Research Findings into Nursing Practice. *Journal of Advanced Nursing.* 12, pp 101-110.

Ifill, C. (1998) One of a kind. *Nursing Times.* pp 14-15.

Incorvaia, D. and Baldwin, S. (1997) Drugs Behind Bars (Part II): A multi-dimensional approach to correctional services settings. *Journal of Substance Misuse for Nursing Health and Social Care.* 2, pp 136-143.

International Association of Forensic Nurses and American Nurses Association (1997) *Scope and Standards of Forensic Nursing Practice.* Washington: American Nurses Publishing.

Jackson, P. (1998) Focus group interviews as a methodology. *Nurse Researcher.* 6(1), pp 72-84.

James, A. (1996) Suicide reduction in medium security. *Journal of Forensic Psychiatry.* pp 406-412.

Jaworowski, S., Nachmias, S. and Zabow, A. (1995) Enforced psychiatric treatment of minors in Israel: The interface between the Mental Health Act and the Youth Law. *Israel Journal of Psychiatry and Related Sciences.* 32(2), pp 114-119.

Jaychuk, G., Manchanda, R. and Galbraith, D.A. (1991) Consent to treatment: Loophole in the Ontario Mental Health Act. *Canadian Journal of Psychiatry.* 36(8), pp 594-596.

Johns, C. and Freshwater, D. (1999) *Transforming Nursing Through Reflective Practice.* Oxford: Blackwell Science.

Joint Prison Service and the National Health Service Executive Working Group (1999) The Future Organisation of Prison Health Care. London: Department of Health.

Jowett, S., Peters, M., Wilson-Barnett, J. and Reynolds, H. (1997) Scope of professional practice - interim report. Unpublished report prepared for UKCC.

Kaye, C. and Franey, A. (1998) *Managing High Security Psychiatric Care.* London: Jessica Kingsley Publications.

Kaye, C. and Franey, A. (1999) About the size of it. *Health Service Journal.* May 1999. Pp 24-25.

Kershaw, C.R.G. (1997) Statistics of Mentally Disordered Offenders in England and Wales. *Home Office Statistical Bulletin.* Sept (20/97)

Killian, M. and Clark, N. (1996) The Nurse. In: Cordess and Cox, (Eds.) *Forensic Psychotherapy; Crime, Psychodynamics and the offender patient,* pp101-106. London: Jessica Kingsley Publications.

Kim, H. (1993) Putting Theory into Practice: Problems and Prospects. *Journal of Advanced Nursing.* 18, pp 1632-1639.

Kim, J.et al. (1998) Racial differences in health status and health behaviours of older adults. *Nursing Research.* Pp 243-250.

King, R. (1994) A Year in Holloway - The Population Survey 1993-1994. London: HMP Holloway.

Kinnear, P.R. and Gray, C.D. (1994) *SPSS for Windows made simple.* London: Erlbaum (UK) Taylor and Francis.

Kinsella, C. and Chaloner, C. (1995) Attitude to treatment and direction of interest of forensic mental health nurses: a comparison with nurses working in other specialities. *Journal of Psychiatric and Mental Health Nursing.* 2(6), pp 351-357.

Kirby S.D and Maguire N.A (1997) Forensic Psychiatric Nursing. In: Thomas, S., Hardy, S. and Cutting, P., (Eds.) *Stuart and Sundeens' Mental Health Nursing: Principles and Practice,* Chap.26, pp 395-409. London: Mosby.

Kirby, S.D. and Pollock, P.H. (1995) The relationship between a medium secure environment and occupational stress in forensic psychiatric nurses. *Journal of Advanced Nursing.* 22, pp 862-867.

Kirk-Smith, M. and McKenna, H. (1998) Psychological concerns in questionnaire research. *Nursing Times.*

Kitchener, N., Wright, I. and Topping-Morris, B. (1992) The Role of The Forensic Nurse. *Nursing Times.* 91(25), pp 11-12.

Kitzinger, J. (1996) Introducing focus groups. In: Mays, N. and Pope, C., (Eds.) *Qualitative Research in Health Care,* Chap.5, 3pp 6-45. London: BMJ Publishing Group.

Kitzinger, S. (1996) Sheila Kitzinger's Letter from Europe: Women Prisoners Freed from Birth Chains: A Successful Campaign. *BIRTH.* 23(3), pp 169-171.

Kitzinger, S. (1997) Sheila Kitzinger's Letter from Europe: How Can We Help Pregnant Women and Mothers in Prison? *BIRTH.* 24(3), pp 197-198.

Kitzinger, S. (1998) The hardest labour of all. *The Guardian.* Newspaper article: 16 Mar 1998.

Kitzinger, S. (1999) Birth in Prison - the rights of the baby. *Practising Midwife.* 2(1), pp 16-18.

Kornreich, J. (1991) Borderlines. *Long Island Voice.* Newspaper article.

Kratzer Worley, N., Drago, L. and Hadley, T. (1990) Improving the physical health-mental health interface for the chronically mentally ill: Could nurse case managers make a difference? *Archives of Psychiatric Nursing*. April 1990. IV (2), pp 108-113.

Krueger R.A (1995) The future of focus groups. *Qualitative Health Research*. 5(4), pp 524-530.

Krueger, R.A. (1994) *Focus Groups: A Practical Guide for Applied Research*. 2nd edn. London: Sage.

Lacey, E.A. (1994) Research Utilisation in Research Practice: A pilot study. *Journal of Advanced Nursing*. 19, pp 987-995.

Lart, R. (1998) The Wessex Project: Meeting the mental health needs of prisoners. *Prison Service Journal*. p 21.

Lart, R. and Payne, S. et al. (1998) Women and Secure Psychiatric Services: a literature review. Report to NHS Centre for Reviews and Dissemination. Bristol University.

Le Var, R. (1996) NVQ's in nursing, midwifery and health. A question of assessment and learning. *Nurse Education Today*. 16(2), pp 85-93.

Lehane, M. and Rees, C. (1996) Alternatives to seclusion in psychiatric care. *British Journal of Nursing*. 5(16), pp 974-979.

Lewin, R.J.P., Ingleton, R., Newens, A.J. and Thompson, D.R. (1998) Adherence to cardiac rehabilitation guidelines: a survey of rehabilitation programmes in the United Kingdom. *British Medical Journal*. 316, pp 1354-1355.

Liebling, H., Chipchase, H. and Velangi, R. (1997) Why do women harm themselves? Surviving Special Hospitals. *Feminism and Psychology*. 7, pp 427-437.

Liebling, H., Chipchase, H. and Velangi, R. (1997) An evaluation of nurse training and support needs: Working with women patients who harm themselves in a Special Hospital. *Issues in Criminological and Legal Psychology*. 29, pp 47-56.

Lipp, A. (1998) An enquiry into a combined approach for nursing ethics. *Nursing Ethics*. 5(2), pp 122-138.

Littlewood, R. and Lipsedge, M. (1995) Ethnic minorities and the psychiatrist. In: Davey, B. et al., (Ed.) *Health and disease*, 2nd revised edn. Pp 50-54. Buckingham: Open University Press.

Longfield, M.D. (1998) Prison Health. Annual Report of The Director of Health Care 1996-97. London: HMSO.

Lovell, K. (1995) User satisfaction with in-patient mental health services. *Journal of Psychiatric and Mental Health Nursing*. 2(3), pp 143-150.

Lygo, R. (1991) Review of the Management of the Prison service. London: HMSO.

Lynch, V. (1993) Forensic nursing: diversity in education and practice. *Journal of Psychosocial Nursing and Mental Health Services*. 31(11), pp 7-14

Lyne, M. (1997) No Bars On Care. *Nursing Standard*. 12(11), p 18.

MacGuire, J.M. (1990) Putting Nursing Research Findings into Practice: Research Utilization as an aspect of the Management of Change. *Journal of Advanced Nursing*. 15,pp 614-620.

Maden, T., Curle, C., Meux, C., Burrow, S. and Gunn, J. (1995) *Treatment & Security Needs of Special Hospital Patients.* London: Whurr Publishers Ltd.

Maeve, M.K. (1997) Nursing practice with incarcerated women: caring within mandated (sic) alienation. *Issues in Mental Health Nursing*. 18(5), pp 495-510.

Maguire N.A (1999) Models of Imperfection. *Health Service Journal*. May 1999. pp20-22.

Mahoney, C. (1997) Managing the risk. *Nursing Times*. 93, pp 73-76.

Mahood, N.J., Colgan, L.M. and Bocus, Y. (1995) Training Needs Analysis of Qualified Nurses. Unpublished report. NHS Trust: Mental Health Services of Salford [Eds.]

Main, T.F. (1957) The Ailment. In: Reprinted In: Main, T.F., (Ed.) *The Ailment And Other Psychoanalytic Essays*, Chap.2, pp 12-35. London: Free Association.

Mak, F.L. (1998) The Development of the Core Curriculum in Psychiatry. *Current Opinion on Psychiatry*. 11(5).

Mangan, P. (1995) Invisible mending ... the skills of a qualified psychiatric nurse can make a real difference to people's lives. *Nursing Times*. 91, pp 66-68.

Mansfield, B. and Matthews, D. (1985) The Components of Job Competence. Bristol: Further Education Staff College.

Mansfield, B. and Mitchell, L. (1996) Towards a Competent Workforce. Hampshire: Gower Publishing Ltd.

Marlowe, M. and Sugarman, P. (1997) ABC of mental health ... Disorders of personality. *British Medical Journal*. p 315.

Marmot, M.G., Aldestein, A.M. and Bulusu, L. (1984) Immigrant Mortality in England and Wales 1970-78: Causes of Death by Country of Birth. London: HMSO.

Marr, J. and Khadim, N. (1993) Meeting the needs of ethnic patients. *Nursing Standard*. 8(3), pp 31-33.

Martin, E. (1989) Prison Medicine. *The Practitioner*. 233, p 805.

Mason, D., Birmingham, L. and Grubin, D. (1997) Substance misuse in remand prisoners: a consecutive case study. *British Medical Journal*. 315, pp 18-21.

Mason, T. and Chandley, M. (1990) Nursing models in a Special Hospital: a critical analysis of efficacity. *Journal of Advanced Nursing*. 15,pp 667-673.

Mason, T. and Patterson, R. (1990) A critical review of the use of Rogers' model within a Special Hospital: a single case study. *Journal of Advanced Nursing*. 15, pp 130-141.

Mason, T. and Chandley, M. (1992) Nursing models in a Special Hospital: cybernetics, hyperreality and beyond. *Journal of Advanced Nursing*. 17, pp 1350-1354.

Mason, T. (1993) Special Hospital seclusion and its clinical variations. *Journal of Clinical Nursing*. 2, pp 95-102.

Mason, T. and Whittington, T. (1995) Seclusion: the use of a stress model to appraise the problem. *Nursing Times*. 91, pp 31-33.

Mason, T. and Mercer, D. (1996) Forensic psychiatric nursing: visions of social control. *Australian New Zealand Journal of Mental Health Nursing*. 5, pp 153-162.

Mason, T. (1998) Tarasoff liability: it's impact for working with patients who threaten others. *International Journal of Nursing Studies*. Pp 109-114.

May Committee (1977) Committee of Inquiry into the United Kingdom Prison Services. London: HMSO.

May, N., Veitch, L., McIntosh, J. and Alexander, M. (1997) *Evaluation of Nurse and Midwife Education in Scotland; 1992 programmes.* Edinburgh: NBS.

Mayne, L. (1998) Women in Special Hospitals. [Personal communication.]

McCann, G. (1996) Speaking terms ... Nurses in forensic institutions could play a major role in reducing their own isolation. *Nursing Times*. 92, p 52

McComish, A.G. and Paterson, B. (1996) The development of forensic services in Scotland 1800-1960. *Psychiatric Care*. 3, pp 153-158.

McEvoy, C. (1995) The report of the summative evaluation of Project 2000 in Northern Ireland. Belfast: NBNI.

McGovern, D. and Cope, R. (1987) First Psychiatric admission rates of first and second generation Afro-Caribbeans. *Social Psychiatry*, 22 pp 139-149

McHugh, A., Wain, I. and West, M. (1995) Mental Health: Handle with care. *Nursing Times*. 91, pp 62-63.

McKenna, H.P. (1995) Dissemination and application of mental health nursing research. *British Journal of Nursing*. 4(21).

McKenzie, K. (1999) Something borrowed from the blues. British Medical Journal, 318, pp 616-617

McKeown, M. and Stowell-Smith, M. (1998) Language, race and forensic psychiatry: Some dilemmas for anti-discriminatory practice. In: Mason, T. and Mercer, D., (Eds.) *Critical Perspectives in Forensic Care: inside out*, Chap.12, pp 188-208. London: McMillan Press Ltd.

McKeown, M. and Mercer, D. (1998) Fallen from Grace: women, power and knowledge. In: Mason, T. and Mercer, D., (Eds.) *Critical Perspectives in Forensic Care: inside out*, Chap.13, pp 209-229. London: McMillan Press Ltd.

McLean, S.A.M. (1989) *A Patient's Right to Know: Information Disclosure, the Doctor and the Law.* Aldershot: Dartmouth.

McLellan, A.T. (1986) "Psychiatric severity" as a predictor of outcome from substance abuse treatment. In: Meyer, R.E., (Ed.) *Psychopathology and addictive disorders..* New York: Guilford Press.

McMillan, I. (1991) Uncertain future ... psychiatric nursing. *Nursing Times.* pp 87, 19.

McMillan, I. (1991) Life after Broadmoor ... being a patient in the top-security Special Hospital. *Nursing Times.* 87, pp 40-41.

McMillan, I. (1994) Dangerous liaisons ... mental health nurses must brush up on their communication skills, according to a Mental Health Foundation report. *Nursing Times.* 90, p 23.

McMillan, I. (1994) Mental Health: Healthy inside ... a scheme at Blakenhurst, a new commercially run prison, could be the shape of things to come for prison nursing. *Nursing Times.* 90, pp 14-15.

McMillan, I. (1994) Solid as a rock ... Tony Butterworth, Chairman of the Mental Health Nursing Review team. *Nursing Times.* p 90.

McMillan, I. (1996) Mental Health: The Three Professors. *Nursing Times.* 92, pp 58-59.

McMillan, I. (1997) Mental Health: Behind bars. *Nursing Times.* 93, pp 34-35.

McMillan, I. (1997) Mental Health: Broadmoor is first among equals. [News]. 93, pp 18-19.

McMillan, I. (1997) Relationships with patients. *Nursing Standard.* 11, pp 22-24.

McMurran, M., Clerkin, P. and Rosenberg, H. (1997) Problems of female patients in a secure psychiatric hospital. *Psychology, Crime and the Law.* p 19.

McNaught, A. (1987) Health Action and Ethnic Minorities. London: Bedford Square Press

Melia, P. (1997) Boundaries and Inter-Relatedness: Practice issues within the Personality Disorder Service. In: Ashworth Hospital Authority, (Ed.) *The Written Submission to the Committee of Inquiry into the Personality Disorder Unit, Ashworth Hospital Authority.*, Ashworth Hospital Authority.

Mental Health Act Commission (1991) *4th Biennial Report 1989-91.* London: HMSO

Mental Health Act Commission (1999) *8th Biennial Report 1997-99.* London: HMSO

Mental Health Foundation (1997) Approaches to Needs Assessment: Commissioning Services for Offenders with Mental Health Problems. 2nd of 6 Monographs. p.32 London: Mental Health Foundation.

Menzies-Lyth, I. (1988) *Containing Anxiety in Institutions: Selected Essays.* London: Free Association.

Mercer, K. (1986) Racism and Transcultural Psychiatry. In Miller, P. Rose, > (eds) The Power of Psychiatry, pp 112-142. Oxford: Blackwell

Metzner, J. (1997) An introduction to Correctional Psychiatry: Part 2. *Journal of the American Academy of Psychiatry and Law.* p 579.

Miller, J. and Messenger, S. (1978) Obstacles to Applying Nursing Research Findings. *American Journal of Nursing.* 8(4), pp 632-634.

Milligan, F. (1998) Refining and assessing competence: the distractions of outcomes and the. *Nursing Education Today.* pp 273-280.

Ministry of Health (1961) Special Hospitals: Report of Working Party. (The Emery Report). London: HMSO.

Ministry of Health (1968) Psychiatric Nursing Today and Tomorrow: Standing Mental Health and Standing Nursing Advisory Committees. Ministry of Health: Central Health Services Council.

Mitchell, D. (1998). Power, professions and evidence based guidelines: Lessons from an organisational case study. *Journal of Nursing Management.* 6, pp 275-280.

Mitchell, L. (1998) Paper presented at the RCN Vocational Qualification Forum Conference. 10 May 1998.

Mohan, D., Scully, P., Collins, C. and Smith, C. (1997). Psychiatric disorder in an Irish female prison. *Criminal Behaviour and Mental Health.* 7, pp 229-235.

Moodley, P, and Thornicroft, G. (1988) Ethnic group and compulsory detention. *Medicine, Science and the Law,* 28 pp 324-328

Moos, R.H. and Houts, P.S. (1968) Assessment of the Social Atmospheres of Psychiatric Wards. *Journal of Abnormal Psychology.* 73(6), pp 595-604.

Moran, T. and Mason, T. (1996) Revisiting the nursing management of the psychopath. *Journal of Psychiatric and Mental Health Nursing.* 3, pp 189-194.

Morgan, D.L. (1995) Why things (sometimes) go wrong in focus groups. *Qualitative Health Research.* 5(4), pp 516-523.

Morison, M. and Moir, J. (1998) The role of computer software in the analysis of qualitative data: efficient clerk. *Journal of Advanced Nursing.* 28(1), pp 106-116.

Morris, S. and Rushton, R. (1993) Self reported suicidal thoughts and behaviours at HMP Holloway. London: HMP Holloway.

Morrison, P. and Burnard, P. (1992) Introduction. In: Burnard, P. and Morrison, P., (Eds.) *Aspects of Forensic Psychiatric Nursing,* Vol. 1. Aldershot: Avebury.

Morrison, P., Burnard, P. and Philips, C. (1996) Patient satisfaction in a forensic unit. *Journal of Mental Health.* 5, pp 369-377.

Morrison, P., Phillips, C. and Burnard, P. (1996) Research In Brief: Staff and patient satisfaction in a forensic unit. *Journal of Psychiatric and Mental Health Nursing.* 3, pp 67-68.

Morse J.N (1992) Strategies for sampling. In: Morse J.N, (Ed.) *Qualitative nursing research*, Chap.8, pp 127-145.

Muir Gray, J.A. (1997) *Evidence based healthcare: how to make health policy and management decisions.* London: Churchill Livingstone.

Murphy, E. (1996) The past and future of Special Hospitals. *Journal of Mental Health UK.* 5, pp 475-482.

Murray, K. (1996) The use of beds in NHS medium secure units in England. *Journal of Forensic Psychiatry.* 7, pp 504-524.

Mussallem, H.K. (1983) International bodies and prison health care. *International Nursing Review.* 30(6), 183-185.

Myco, F. (1980) Nursing Research Information: Are nurse educators and practitioners seeking it out? *Journal of Advanced Nursing.* 6, 51-58.

Naish, J. (1997) Leadership. So where's the evidence? *Nursing Times.* 93, 64-66.

National Health Service (1977) National Health Service Act. London: HMSO.

National Health Service Executive (1994) Black Mental Health- A dialogue for change. Mental Health Task Force. Leeds:NHS Executive.

National Health Service Executive (1996) Promoting Clinical Effectiveness: A framework for action in and through the NHS. Leeds: NHS Executive.

Newbold (1996) An evaluation of the role of the nurse practitioner. *Nursing Times.* 92, pp 45-46.

NHS Executive (1998) Health Service Circular: Widening access to nursing and midwifery education and training. HSC/1998/182. London: NHS Executive.

NHS Executive (1998) Modernising Mental Health Services. London: NHS Executive.

NHS Executive North West Regional Office (1998) Core Competencies for Mental Health Workers. Report of working group. Warrington: NHS Executive.

Niskala, H. (1986) Competencies and skills required by nurses working in forensic areas. *Western Journal of Nursing Research.* 8, 400-413.

Niskala, H. (1987) Conflicting convictions: nurses in forensic settings. *Canadian Journal of Psychiatric Nursing.* 28, pp 10-14.

Noak, J. (1995) Care of people with psychopathic disorder. *Nursing Standard.* 9, pp 30-32.

Noak, J. (1997) Assessment of the risks posed by people with mental illness. *Nursing Times*. 93, pp 34-36.

Norman, A. and Parrish, A. (1999) Prison health care: work environment and the nursing role. *British Journal of Nursing*. 8(10), pp 653-656.

Northern Ireland Office (1998) A Commentary on Northern Ireland Crime Statistics 1997. Belfast: The Stationery Office.

Nursing Board for Scotland (1995) Competence to practice. A literature review on competence to practice. Edinburgh: NBS.

Nursing Times (1997) UKCC urged to resolve prison nursing conflict. *Nursing Times*. 93 (22), p 7.

O'Hanlon, M. and Andrews, D. (1997) Occupational Standards - A Framework for Clinical Effectiveness? Liverpool: The Royal Liverpool University Hospitals.

O'Sullivan, J. (1998) Woman prisoner pleads to keep new-born girl. *The Independent*. Newspaper article: 5 Nov 1998.

Office for National Statistics (1997) Psychiatric morbidity among prisoners in England and Wales.

Ogden, J. (1995) Labour chains ... is a prisoner in the throes of labour such a security risk she needs to be kept in handcuffs? *Nursing Times*. 91, p 18.

Okwuosah, A. (1996) Health Status of Women in Nigerian Prisons. In: Squires, N. and Stobl, J., (Eds.) *Healthy Prisons: a vision for the future. Report of the International Conference on Health Prisons.*, pp 223-227. Liverpool: University of Liverpool - Department of Public Health.

Orem, D. (1985) *Nursing: Concepts of Practice*. New York: McGraw-Hill.

Osbourne, O.II. (1995) Jailed mothers: further explorations in public sector nursing. *Journal of Psychosocial Nursing and Mental Health Services*. 33, pp 22-28.

Papadopoulos, I. and Alleyne, J. (1995) The need for nursing and midwifery programmes of education to address the health care needs of minority ethnic groups. *Nurse Education Today*. Apr 1995. 15(2), pp 140-144.

Parkes, J. (1996) Control and restraint training: A study of its effectiveness in a medium secure psychiatric unit. *Journal of Forensic Psychiatry*. 7, pp 525-534.

Parrish, A. (1996) Should the NHS take over the prison service? *British Journal of Nursing*. p 1226.

Paterson, B., Tringham, C., McComish, A. and Waters, S. (1997) Managing aggression and violence: a legal perspective on the use of force. *Psychiatric Care*. 4, pp 128-131.

Paterson, B., Leadbetter, D. and McComish, A. (1997) De-escalation in the management of aggression and violence. *Nursing Times*. 93, pp 58-61.

Paterson, B., Leadbetter, D. and McComish, A. (1998) Restraint and sudden death from asphyxia. *Nursing Times*. 94, pp 62-64.

Paterson, B and Leadbetter D (1999) Managing Physical Violence in Turnbull J and Patterson B, Aggression and Violence Approaches to effective management. London: Macmillan

Pegram, E.G. (1997) Do nurses or any other health care staff working in the Prison Health Care Service face a conflict of interests in their role as carers against their role as custodians?, and do any of their actions breach the United Kingdom Central Council for Nursing, Midwifery and Health Visiting Code of Professional Conduct? University of Bradford. BSc Professional Practice in Health Care. [Unpublished Dissertation]

Pensker, H. (1983) Addicted patients in hospital psychiatric units. *Psychiatric Annals*. 13, pp 619-623.

Peternelj-Taylor, C. and Johnson, R.L (1996) Custody and Caring: clinical placement of student nurses in a forensic setting. *Perspectives in Psychiatric Care*. 32(44), pp 23-29.

Peternelj-Taylor, C. (1998) Forbidden love: sexual exploitation in the forensic milieu. *Journal of Psychosocial Nursing and Mental Health Services*. 6, p 23.

Peternelj-Taylor, C.A. and Hufft, A.G. (1997) *Forensic Psychiatric Nursing*. Lippincott Raven Publishers.

Peternelj Taylor, C.A. and Johnson, R.L. (1995) Serving time: psychiatric mental health nursing in corrections. *Journal of Psychosocial Nursing and Mental Health Services*. 33(8), pp 12-19.

Peters, R.H. and Hills, H.A. (1993) Inmates with co-occurring substance abuse and mental health disorders. In: Steadman, H.J. and Cocozza, J.J., (Eds.) *Providing services for offenders with mental illness and related disorders in prisons*. pp 160-211. Washington D.C.: The National Coalition for the Mentally Ill in the Criminal Justice System.

Pettengill, M., Gillies, D. and Lark, C. (1994) Factors encouraging and discouraging the use of Research Findings. *Journal of Nursing Scholarship*. Summer. 26(2), pp 143-147.

Phillips, M.S. (1983) "Forensic psychiatric - nurses" attitudes revealed. *Dimensions*. 60(9), pp 42-43.

Pillette, C. et al. (1995) Therapeutic management of helping boundaries. 33(1), pp 40-47.

Pitt, R. (1993) Who cares?... Consigning people with mental illness or learning disabilities to prison. *Nursing Times*. 89, pp 27-29.

Polit, D.F. and Hungler, B.P. (1989) *Essentials of nursing research: methods, appraisals and utilisation*. 2nd Edition edn. Philadelphia: J.B. Lippincott.

Polit, D.F. and Hungler, B.P. (1993) *Essentials of Nursing Research: appraisal and utilisation.* Philadelphia: J.B. Lippincot Company.

Prins, H. (1991) Big, black and dangerous? Report of the Committee of Inquiry into the death in Broadmoor Hospital of Orville Blackwood and a Review of the deaths of two other Afro Caribbean patients.

Prins H and Swan M(1998) Independent inquiries into homicides. *Psychiatric Care* 5 (3) pp 112-117

Prison Libraries Group (1998) Prison Libraries Training Pack. London: Home Office.

Rampton Hospital Authority (1998) *The Forensic Directory. National Health and Private Forensic Facilities in The United Kingdom.* 3rd edn. Rampton Hospital Authority, Social Work Department.

Ramsbotham, Sir D. (1999) Paper presented at the RCN Nurses working in prison Conference. 12 May 1999.

Ranney, M.H. (1850) On insane foreigners. *American Journal of Insanity.* 7,p 53. Cited in Farrington A (1993). *British Journal of Nursing*, 2(16) , pp 805-809

Rassool, G.H. (1995) The Health Status and Health Care of Ethno-Cultural Minorities in the United Kingdom: an agenda for action. *Journal of Advanced Nursing.* 21(2), pp 199-201.

Redfern (1997) Reactions to nurses' expanding practice. *Nursing Times.* 93(32), pp 45-47.

Reed, J. (1992) The Academic and Research Base. The Reports of the Academic Development and Research Advisory Groups. Vol. 4. pp 10-39. London: Department of Health, Home Office.

Reed, J. (1992) Review of Health and Social Services for the Mentally Disordered Offenders and others Requiring Similar Services. Volume 3. pp 84-129. Department of Health, Home Office.

Reed, J. (1994) Report of the Department of Health and Home Office Working Group on Psychopathic Disorder. London: Department of Health, Home Office.

Reed, J. and Lyne, M. (1997) The quality of health care in prison: results of a year's programme of semistructured inspections. *British Medical Journal.* 315, pp 1420-1424.

Reeder, D. and Meldman, L. (1991) Conceptualizing psychosocial nursing in the jail setting. *Journal of Psychosocial Nursing and Mental Health Services.* 29(8), pp 40-47.

Rehman, H. and Walker, E. (1995) Researching black and minority ethnic groups. *Health Education Journal.* 54(4), pp 489-500.

Repper, J., Brooker, C. and Repper, D. (1995) Serious mental health problems: policy changes. *Nursing Times.* 91, pp 29-31.

Repper, J., Perkins, R., Owen, S., Deighton, D. and Robinson, J. (1996) Evaluating services for women with serious and ongoing mental health problems: developing an appropriate research method. *Journal of Psychiatric and Mental Health Nursing.* 3(1), pp 39-46.

Repper, J. and Perkins, A. (1998) A tricky act. *Nursing Times.*

Reynolds, J. and Smartt, U. (1996) Prison Policy and Practice: Selected papers from 35 years of the Prison Service Journal. *Prison Service Journal.*

Richman, J. (1998) The ceremonial and moral order of a ward for psychopaths. In: Mason, T. and Mercer, D., (Eds.) *Critical perspectives in forensic care*, Chap.10, pp 146-170. London: McMillan Press Ltd.

Ricketts, T. (1998) Single case research in mental health. *Nursing Times.*

Right Hon Lord Justice Woolf and his Honour Judge Stephen Tumin (1991) Prison Disturbances - Apr 1990. London: HMSO.

Robinson, D., Reed, V. (1996) Measuring Forensic Psychiatric and Mental Health Nursing Interventions. Developments in Nursing and Health Care Series 11 Aldershot: Avebury

Robinson, D., Reed, V. and Lange, A. (1996) Developing risk assessment scales in forensic psychiatric care. *Psychiatric Care* 3(4) : pp 146-152

Robinson, D. (1996) Developing the contribution of research in nursing practice, *Psychiatric Care.* 3(2): pp 45-50

Robinson, D. (1998) Forensic Care: new opportunities and challenges. *Psychiatric Care* 5(4): p 121

Robinson, D. and McGregor A. (1998) The lost vision of nursing. *Psychiatric Care* 5(4): pp 126-129

Robinson, D. and Kettles, A. (1998) The emerging profession of forensic nursing: myth or reality? *Psychiatric Care.* 5(6), pp 214-218.

Robinson, D., Whyte, L. and Fidler I (1997) Quality of life measures in a high security environment. *Nursing Standard.* 11, pp 34-37.

Rogers, A. and Faulkner, A. (1987) *A place of safety.* London: MIND

Rogers, P. (1995) Restraint debate continues ... "Handle with care". *Nursing Times.* 91, p 24.

Rogers, P. and Topping-Morris, B. (1996) Prison and the role of the forensic mental health nurse. *Nursing Times.* 92(31), pp 32-34.

Rogers, P. and Topping-Morris, B. (1997) Clinical supervision for forensic mental health nurses. *Nursing Management: The Nursing Standard Journal for Nurse Leaders.* 4, pp 13-15.

Rolfe, G. (1998) The theory practice gap in nursing: From research-based practice to practitioner based research. *Journal of Advanced Nursing.* 28(3), pp 672-679.

Rooney, J. (1998) Safety measures. *Health Service Journal.* p 108.

Rose, K., Waterman, H. and Tullo, A. (1997) The extended role of the nurse: reviewing the implications for practice. *Clinical Effectiveness in Nursing.* 1(1), pp 31-37.

Rosenberg, W. and Donald, A. (1995) Evidence based medicine: an approach to clinical problem-solving. *British Medical Journal .* 310, pp 1122-1126.

Rowden, R. (1997) No descent into anarchy at the Special Hospitals. [Interview by Ian McMillan]. *Nursing Standard.* 11, p 12.

Royle, J. and Blythe, J. (1998) Promoting research utilisation in nursing: the role of the individual, organisation and environment. *Evidence Based Nursing.* July 98. 1(3).

Russell, J.H. and Kettles, A.M. (1996) User views of a forensic service. *Psychiatric Care.* 3, pp 98-104.

Rwegellera, G.G.C. (1977) Psychiatric Morbidity among West Africans and West Indians living in London. *Psychological Medicine.* 7, pp 317-329

Rwegellera, G.G.C. (1980) Differential use of psychiatric services by West Africans and West Indians and English in London. *British Journal of Psychiatry,* 137, pp 428-432

Ryan, D. (1997) Ambiguity in Nursing: The person and the organisation as contrasting sources of meaning. In: Tilley, S., (Ed.) *The Mental Health Nurse: Views of practice and education.* Oxford: Blackwell Science.

Ryan, T. (1994) The risk business ... supervision as a solution to problems involving mentally ill people in the community. *Nursing Management: The Nursing Standard Journal for Nurse Leaders.* 1, pp 9-11.

Ryries, R.et al. (1998) A survey of psychiatric nursing practice in two inner city acute admission wards. *Journal of Advanced Nursing.* pp 848-854.

Sackett, D.L.et al. (1996) Evidence based medicine: What it is and what it isn't. *British Medical Journal.* Jan 96. 312(13), pp 71-72.

Safer, D. (1987) Substance abuse by young adult chronic patients. *Hospital and Community Psychiatry.* 38, pp 511-514.

Sainsbury Centre for Mental Health (1997) Pulling Together. The Future Roles and Training of Mental Health Staff. London: Sainsbury Centre for Mental Health.

Sakinofsky, I. (1997) Review: Risk for suicide is increased for most mental disorders where patients require treatment in a hospital setting. Evidence Based Medicine. Sept/Oct. Unpublished.

Sargant, A. (1998) An unacademic response: psychiatric nursing. Unpublished.

Savage, L. and McKeown, M (1997)   Towards a new model of practice for a high dependency unit. *Psychiatric Care*. p 186.

Scales, C., Mitchell, J. and Smith, R. (1993) Survey report on forensic nursing. *Journal of Psychosocial Nursing and Mental Health Services*. 31(11), pp 39-44.

Schafer, P. (1997)   When a client develops an attraction: successful resolution versus boundary violation. *Journal of Psychiatric and Mental Health Nursing*. 4, pp 203-211.

Scott, E.M. (1997) A prison and a nursing home: any similarities? *International Journal of Offender Therapy and Comparative Criminology*. 41, pp 298-310.

Scott, L. and Blantern, S. (1998) Mothers and babies within the prison system. *British Journal of Midwifery*. (August).

Scottish Home and Health Department (1984) Mental Health (Scotland) Act. Edinburgh: Scottish Home and Health Department.

Scottish Office (1998) Prison Statistics Scotland 1997. Edinburgh: Scottish Office.

Scottish Office (1999) Towards a healthier Scotland. Edinburgh: The Stationery Office

Scottish Office (1999)   Health and Social Work and Related Services for Mentally Disordered Offenders in Scotland. A Consultation Paper. Scottish Office: Department of Health.

Scottish Office (1995) Mental Health Records; A good practice statement. CRAG working group on mental illness. Edinburgh: National Health Service in Scotland.

Scottish Office (1997) Designed to care. Department of Health. Edinburgh. The Scottish Office

Scottish Prison Service (undated) Act and Care. Suicide Risk Management Strategy. Edinburgh; Scottish Prison Service

Scrutiny Team (1990)   Report on an Efficiency Scrutiny of the Prison Medical Service. Volumes 1 and 2. London: Directorate of the Prison Medical Service.

Senior, J. (1998) Doctor's orders: the mentally disordered in prison. In: Mason, T. and Mercer, D., (Eds.) *Critical perspectives in forensic care: inside out*, Chap.14, pp 230-243. London: McMillan Press Ltd.

Sensky, T., Hughes, T. and Hirsch, S. (1991) Compulsory psychiatric treatment in the community. A controlled study of compulsory community treatment with extended leave under the Mental Health Act: special characteristics of patients treated and impact of treatment. *British Journal of Psychiatry*. 158, pp 792-799.

Shasidharan, S.P. (1988) Towards an Anti-Racist Psychiatry. Paper given at a conference on Black perspectives on Mental Health Care, London

Shepherd, G. (1984) *Institutional Care and Rehabilitation*. London: Longman.

Shuttleworth, M. (1993) Articulating the competence movement and professional formation. Leicester: De Montfort University. Paper presented at Conference at De Montfort University.

Siegel, S. and Castellan Jr, N.J. (1988) *Non-parametric statistics for the behavioural sciences.* 2nd edn. Singapore: McGraw Hill.

Sim, J. (1998) Collecting and analysing qualitative data: issues raised by the focus group. *Journal of Advanced Nursing.* pp 345-352.

Singer, P. (1993) *Practical Ethics.* 2nd edn. Cambridge: Cambridge University Press.

Small, M. (1995) Perinatal and neonatal mortality in ethnic minorities. *Modern Midwife.* 5(4), pp 29-31.

Smith, A. and Humphreys, M. (1997) Characteristics of in-patients transferred to a locked ward in a Scottish psychiatric hospital. *Health Bulletin.* P 82.

Smith, C.D. (1998) Assessing health needs in women's prisons. *Prison Service Journal.* pp 118, 22-24.

SNMAC (1999) The role of the mental health nurse in the provision of modern Mental Health Acute Care. Report of the Standing Nursing and Midwifery Advisory Committee. September 1999.

Soloff, P.H. and Turner, S.M. (1981) Patterns of seclusion: a prospective study. *Journal of Nervous and Mental Diseases,* 169 (19), pp 37-44

Squires, N. and Stobl, J. (1996) Healthy Prisons: a vision for the future. Report of the International Conference on Health Prisons. pp 220-222. Liverpool: University of Liverpool - Department of Public Health.

Stevens, R. (1993) When Your Clients Are In Jail. *Nursing Forum.* 28(4), pp 4-5.

Stockwell, F. (1972) The Unpopular Patient. 1st edn, Volume 2. London: Royal College of Nursing.

Storey, L., Dale, C. and Martin, E. (1997) Social therapy: a developing model of care for people with personality disorders. *Nursing Times research.* 2(3), pp 210-218.

Storey, L. (1998) Functional analysis and occupational standards: their role in curriculum development. *Nurse Education Today* . 18, pp 3-11.

Storey, L, Woods, P., Bradshaw, R. and Landsberg G (1999) NYPD Blues. *Mental Health and Learning Disabilities Care.* 2(11) pp 371-372

Storey, L. (1999) Mental Health Nursing in Roskilde County Denmark. http://www.graduate research.com

Storey, L. and Dale, C. (1998) Meeting the needs of patients with severe personality disorders. *Mental Health Practice.* 1(5), pp 20-26.

Storey, L. and Dale, C. (1998) Nursing in secure environments. *Psychiatric Care*. 5(4), pp 122-123.

Storey, L., O'Kell, S. and Day, M. (1995) Utilising occupational standards as a complement to nurse education. Leeds: NHS Executive.

Street, A. (1995) *Nursing Replay: Researching nursing culture.* Melbourne: Churchill Livingstone.

Street, A. and Walsh, C. (1998) Nursing assessments in New Zealand mental health. *Journal of Advanced Nursing*. 27, pp 553-559.

Street, A.F. and Walsh, C. (1994) The legislation of the therapeutic role: implications for the practice of community mental health nurses using the New Zealand Mental Health (Compulsory Assessment and Treatment) Act of 1992. *Australian New Zealand Journal of Mental Health Nursing*. 3, pp 39-44.

Strong, S. (1997) Caught short. *Nursing Times*. 93, pp 38-40.

Strong, S. (1998) Sentenced. *Nursing Times*.

Sturm, R. and McCulloch, J. (1998) Mental health and substance abuse benefits in carve-out plans and the Mental Health Parity Act of 1996. *Journal of Health Care Finance*. 24, pp 82-92.

Swidler, R.N. and Tauriello, J.V. (1995) New York State's Community Mental Health Reinvestment Act. *Psychiatric Services*. 46(5), pp 496-500.

Swinton, M. and Smith, S. (1997) Costs of physical health care for self-injuring patients. *Psychiatric Bulletin*. 21, pp 483-541.

Symonds, B. (1998) The philosophical and sociological context of mental health care legislation. *Journal of Advanced Nursing*. 27, pp 946-954.

Tadd, W. (1997) How practitioners interpret and use the UKCC code of professional conduct for nurses, midwives and health visitors in their practice. [Unpublished post doctoral research proposal].

Tarbuck P (1998) Health care in prisons: agenda for change. *Mental Health Practice*. 1(7), pp 10-12.

Tarbuck, P. (1992) Use and abuse of control and restraint. *Nursing Standard*. 6, pp 30-32.

Tarbuck, P. (1992) Ethical standards and human rights. *Nursing Standard*. 7, pp 27-30.

Tarbuck, P. (1994) *Buying Forensic Mental Health Nursing: A Guide for Purchasers.* London: Royal College of Nursing.

Tarbuck, P. and Thompson, T. (1995) Defining and treating challenging behaviour. *Nursing Standard*. 9, pp 30-33.

Tarbuck, P. and Thirkettle, B. (1996) Towards a language for mental health nursing... Read Code Thesaurus. *Psychiatric Care*. 3, pp 59-64.

Tarbuck, P. (1996) A review of the literature concerning Medium Secure Mental Health Services. Prepared for the HAS visit to the North West Region Health Authority. [Unpublished work].

Tate, C.W. (1996) All talk and no action ... Gap between making recommendations and implementing policy on ethnic minorities in the health service. *Nursing Management.* 3(5), p 7.

Taylor, P.J., Maden, A. and Jones, D. (1996) Long-term medium-security hospital units: A service gap of the 1990s? *Criminal Behaviour and Mental Health.* 6, pp 213-229.

Taylor, P.J., Leese, M., Williams, D., Butwell, M., Daly, R. and Larkin, E. (1998) Mental disorder and violence: A special (high security) hospital study. *British Journal of Psychiatry.* 172, pp 218-226.

Tennant, A. and Hughes, G. (1997) Issues in nursing care for patients with severe personality disorders. *Mental Health Practice.* p 16.

Teplin, L.A., Abram, K.M. and McClelland, G.M. (1997) Mentally disordered women in jail: Who receives services? *American Journal of Public Health.* 87, pp 604-609.

The Foundation of Nursing Studies (1996) Reflection for Action. London: The Foundation of Nursing Studies.

The Howard League (1995) "I thought babies weren't prisoners. Why are they being deprived?" The Howard League Information: Prison Mother and Baby Units. Pp 1-12. London: The Howard League.

The Mental Health Foundation (1998) Commissioning Services for Offenders with Mental Health Problems. London: The Mental Health Foundation.

The Standard Nursing Midwifery Advisory Committee (1998) The Role of the Mental Health Nurse in the Provision of Modern Mental Health Acute Care. [Unpublished work].

Thomas, B. (1995) Caught in the frontline ... Concern is growing about the widespread use of illicit drugs by patients in psychiatric wards. *Nursing Times.* 91, pp n38-39.

Thomas, L., McColl, E., Cullum, N., Rousseau, N., Soutter, J., Brennand, C. and Steen, N. (1998) Systematic review of the effectiveness of guidelines in nursing and professions allied to medicine. Final report. University of Newcastle upon Tyne - Centre for Health Services Research.

Thomson, L. (1997) The state hospital survey- a description of psychiatric patients in conditions of special security in Scotland. *Journal of Forensic Psychiatry.* p284.

Thomson, M.A. (1998) Closing the gap between nursing research and practice. *Evidence Based Nursing.* Jan 98. 1(1).

Topping-Morris, B. (1992) An historical and personal view of forensic nursing services. In: Morrison, P. and Burnard, P., (Eds.) *Aspects of Forensic Psychiatric Nursing,* Chap.1, pp 2-44. Aldershot: Avebury.

Topping-Morris, B. and McHugh, A. (1995) No place for restraint in care ... "Handle with care". *Nursing Times.* 91, pp 22-24.

Topping-Morris, B. (1997) 'Nurse 97' Awards. Humanising a hidden service ... Barry Topping-Morris (Joint recipient of the 'Nurse 97' Mental Health Award). *Nursing Standard.* 12, pp 20-21.

Travers, R. and Aiyegbusi, A. (1998) A Clinical Paradigm for Women's Services. First draft. [Unpublished work]. Ashworth Hospital Authority.

Treneman, A. (1997) Which of the two sides will be left holding the baby after the battle of the bulge? *The Independent.* Newspaper article: 27 Sep 1997.

Tucker-Allen, S., Williams, D.D. and Wisneski, S.M. (1994) Health care of women in prison: an overview. *ABNF Journal.* 5, pp 52-57.

Twinn, S. (1998) An analysis of the effectiveness of focus groups as a method of qualitative data. *Journal of Advanced Nursing.*

UKCC (1989) Professional Competencies - Rule 18a. London: UKCC.

UKCC (1992) Scope of Professional Practice. London: UKCC.

UKCC (1992) Standards for Administration of Medicines. London: UKCC.

UKCC (1994) The Midwife's Code of Practice. - London: UKCC.

UKCC (1996) Position Statement on Clinical Supervison for Nursing and Health Visiting. London: UKCC.

UKCC (1996) Guidelines for Professional Practice. London: UKCC.

UKCC (1996) Reporting Misconduct - Information for employers and managers. London: UKCC.

UKCC (1996) Issues arising from Professional Conduct Complaints. London: UKCC.

UKCC (1997) PREP - Specialist practice: Consideration of issues relating to embracing nurse practitioners and clinical nurse specialists. Dec 1997 edn, London: UKCC.

UKCC (1998) Code of Professional Conduct. London: UKCC.

UKCC (1998) Guidelines for Records and Record Keeping. London: UKCC.

UKCC (1998) Scope in Practice. London: UKCC.

UKCC (1998) PREP and You. London: UKCC.

UKCC (1998) Guidelines for Mental Health and Learning Disabilities Nursing. London: UKCC.

UKCC (1998) Making a Complaint. London: UKCC.

UKCC (1999) Interim Report of Commission For Education. London: UKCC.

University of Central Lancashire and Ashworth Hospital Authority (1997) Framework of Occupational Standards. [Unpublished work]. University of Central Lancashire.

Van-Wynen, E.A., Peternelj-Taylor, C., Herzling, C. and Koson, C. (1994) Nurses in forensic nursing. *Journal of Psychosocial Nursing and Mental Health Services*. 32, p 10.

Vaughan, B. and Edwards, M.C. (1995) Interface between Research and Practice. Kings Fund Centre.

Veeramah, V. (1995) A study to identify the attitudes and needs of qualified staff concerning the use of research findings in clinical practice within mental health care settings. *Journal of Advanced Nursing*. 22, pp 855-861.

Vestergaard, J. (1994) The Danish Mental Health Act of 1989: Psychiatric discretion and the new legalism. *International Journal of Law and Psychiatry*. 17(2), pp 191-210.

Vousden, M. (1998) The highway code. *Nursing Times*. pp31-32.

Walczak, J.R., MacGuire, D.B. and Haisfield, M.G. (1994) A survey of research related activities and perceived barriers to research utilisation among professional oncology nurses. *Oncology Nursing Forum*. 21(4), pp 710-715.

Walker, N. (1968) Crime and punishment in Britain: The penal system in theory, law and practice. Edinburgh: Edinburgh University Press.

Walker, N. (1991) Dangerous mistakes. *British Journal of Psychiatry*. 158, 7pp 52-757.

Walsh, E.C.L. (1998) An Exploration of Nurses' Perceptions of Working in a Male Prison. King's College, London. MSc in Nursing. [Unpublished Dissertation]

Walsh, M. and Ford, P. (1989) *Nursing Rituals, Research and Rational Action*. Oxford: Butterworth-Heinemann Ltd.

Walsh, M.P. (1998) What is evidence? A critical view for nursing. *Clinical Effectiveness in Nursing*. 2, pp 86-93.

Walton, H. (1998) The Background and Significance of the Core Curriculum in Psychiatry. *Current Opinion in Psychiatry*. 11(5).

Warner, L. (1997) Mental health: Don't just role over and die. *Nursing Times*. 93, pp 30-31.

Warren, J. and Beadsmoore, A. (1997) Preventing violence on mental health wards. *Nursing Times*. 93, pp 47-48.

Warring, T. (1996) Prisoners with diabetes: do they receive appropriate care? *Nursing Times*. 92, pp 38-39.

Waterman, H. (1998) Embracing ambiguities and valuing ourselves: issues of validity in action research. *Journal of Advanced Nursing*.

Waters, J. (1995) No way out ... the rise in prison suicides. *Nursing Times*. 91, pp 20-21.

Watson, C. (1999) Caring for the Mentally Disordered Offender: Perspectives from Scotland. Paper presented at the RCN 1st Annual Conference in Forensic Health Care Proceedings: 27 May 1999.

Watson, C. and Kirby, S. (1999) A Two Nation Perspective on Issues of Practice and Provision for Professionals Caring for Mentally Disordered Offenders. In: Robinson, D. and Kettles, A., (Eds.) *Forensic Nursing and Multi-Disciplinary Care of the Mentally Disordered Offender*. London: Jessica Kingsley Publishers. [In Press].

Watson, H. (1990) Mental Health: Caught between two cultures ... psychiatric care for people from ethnic minorities. *Nursing Times*. 86(39), pp 66-68.

Webb, C. and McKenzie, J. (1993) Where are we now? Research mindedness in the 1990's. *Journal of Clinical Nursing*. 2, 129-133.

Weiss, R.D. (1992) The role of psychopathology in the transition from drug use to abuse and dependence. In: Glantz, M. and Pickens, R., (Eds.) *Vulnerability to drug abuse*. Washington DC: American Psychological Association.

Werlin, E.L. and O'Brien, E. (1984) Attitude change and a prison health care experience. *Journal of Nursing Education*. 23(9), pp 393-397.

West, S. (1996) Head lice and the Mental Health Act: A case in law and ethics. *Professional Leader*. 3, pp 13-15.

Weston E.T (1981) A comparative study of nursing in Scottish and Danish prisons. *Nursing Times*. Feb 81. Pp 376-378.

White, A. and Johnson, M. (1998) The complexities of nursing research with men. *International Journal of Nursing Studies*. pp 41-48.

White, D. (1996) A balancing act: Mental health policymaking in Quebec. *International Journal of Law and Psychiatry*. 19(3-4), pp 289-307.

White, G. and Thomson, A. (1995) Anonymized focus groups as a research tool for health professionals. *Qualitative Health Research*. 5(2), pp 256-261.

White, P. and Iqbal, P. (1998) Revised projections of long term trends in the prison population to 2005. *Home Office Statistical Bulletin*. (2/98, Jan).

White, P. and Woodbridge, J. (1998) The prison population in 1997. *Home Office Statistical Bulletin*. (5/98, Mar).

White, S.J. (1997) Evidence-based practice and nursing: the new panacea? *British Journal of Nursing*. 6, pp 175-178.

Whyte, J.M. and Gajos, M.A. (1996) A study of nurses' knowledge of the UKCC Code of Conduct. *Nursing Standard*. 10(47), pp 35-37.

Whyte, L. (1997) Forensic nursing: a review of concepts and definitions. *Nursing Standard*. 11, pp 46-47.

Whyte, W.F. (1955) *Street corner society.* Chicago: University of Chicago. In Rolfe, G. (1998) The theory practice gap in nursing: From research-based practice to practitioner based research. *Journal of Advanced Nursing.* 28(3), 672-679.

Williams, K. (1996) Editorial comment: Take a balanced view. *Nursing Standard.* 10 12.

Wilmott, Y. (1997) Prison nursing: the tension between custody and care. *British Journal of Nursing.* 6(6) p 333-336.

Wilson, J. (1993) Childbearing within the prison system. *Nursing Standard.* 7, pp 25-28.

Wilson, J.S. and Leasure, R. (1991) Cruel and unusual punishment: the health care of women in prison. *Nurse Practice.* 16(2), pp 32-39.

Wilson, M. (1993) *Mental Health and Britain's Black Communities.* London: Kings Fund

WISH (Women in Special Hospitals) (1999) Defining Gender Issues: Redefining Women's Services.

Wood, J. (1993) Reform of the Mental Health Act 1983: An effective tribunal system. *British Journal of Psychiatry.* 162, pp 14-22.

Woodrow, P. (1996) Exploring confidentiality in nursing practice. *Nursing Standard.* 10, 38-42.

Woods, P. and Mason, T. (1997) Twenty years of admissions to a Special Hospital. *Psychiatric Care.* 4, pp 22-25.

Wool, R.J. (1992) Nursing Service for Prisoners: Policy Statement. London: Directorate of Health Care.

Wool, R.J. (1993) First Report of the Director of Health Care for Prisoners. London: Directorate of Health Care.

World Health Organisation (1988) Learning To Work Together For Health. Report of a WHO study group on multi-professional education for health personnel: a team approach. Switzerland: WHO.

Worley, N.K., Drago, L. and Hadley, T. (1990) Improving the physical health-mental health interface for the chronically mentally ill: could nurse case managers make a difference? *Archives of Psychiatric Nursing.* 4(2), pp 108-113.

Yates, S. (1994) Promoting mental health behind bars. *Nursing Standard.* 8, pp 18-21.

Yee, B.W.K. and Weaver, G.D. (1994) Ethnic minorities and health promotion: developing a "culturally competent" agenda. *Generations.* Spring. 18(1), pp 39-44.